WATER

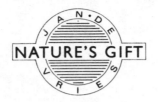

NATURE'S GIFT

Water

JAN DE VRIES

MAINSTREAM
PUBLISHING

First published in 1990 by
MAINSTREAM PUBLISHING CO. (EDINBURGH) LTD
7 Albany Street
Edinburgh EH1 3UG

ISBN 1 85158 346 7 (cloth)
ISBN 1 85158 341 6 (paper)

British Library Cataloguing in Publication Data
De Vries, Jan
  Nature's gift of water.
  1. Medicine. Hydrotherapy
  I. Title
  615.853

  ISBN 1-85158-346-7
  ISBN 1-85158-341-6 pbk

Typeset in 10½/12 Palatino
Reproduced from disc by Polyprint, 48 Pleasance, Edinburgh, EH8 9TJ
Printed and bound in Great Britain by Billings & Sons, Worcester

Contents

Books available from the same author in the
By Appointment Only series:

Stress and Nervous Disorders (sixth impression)

Multiple Sclerosis (third impression)

Traditional Home and Herbal Remedies (third impression)

Arthritis, Rheumatism and Psoriasis (fourth impression)

Do Miracles Exist?

Neck and Back Problems (fifth impression)

Migraine and Epilepsy (third impression)

Cancer and Leukaemia (second impression)

Viruses, Allergies and the Immune System (second impression)

Realistic Weight Control

Available from the same author in the
Nature's Gift series:

Body Energy

Also available from the same author:

Who's Next?

Come back, come back, 'tis Nature bids you come,
Come back once more to tarn and tangled wood,
Come back to glen, and stream, and torrent flood;
Come back, and 'mid the woodlands make your home.
                                        (Samuel Waddington)

1

Water for Life

Water, water, every where
and all the boards did shrink;
Water, water every where
Nor any drop to drink.

　　　　　　　　(Coleridge — *The Ancient Mariner*)

SOME OF MY FONDEST memories of my years at primary
school concern story time and I remember once hearing a
story about a shipwreck. The ship's crew had taken to the
lifeboats and after drifting aimlessly for several days their
supply of drinking water was getting dangerously low.
Water rations were curtailed to the bare minimum as the
survivors were well aware that without fresh water they
would not stand a chance of staying alive until their
rescuers showed up. To a young impressionable mind such
as mine, the sailors' anxiety seemed unwarranted because,
after all, they were drifting in a wide expanse of water. At
that age one may be excused for not realising that none of
this water could fulfil their needs. It is so easily taken for
granted that we merely have to turn on the tap and water

will pour out. Thus we tend to forget that water is a vital elixir of life, without which we would be in dire trouble. Water is not only important for drinking, but it also proves its value in many forms of remedial application. Indeed, we can use water as a life-saver, but only if this water is pure and natural.

Magnetic fields surrounding the earth cause falling raindrops to fragment into spray and this phenomenon 'activates' water. This active water makes minerals soluble. Water is of the greatest importance to our existence. Without water not only would the land be barren and any form of agriculture impossible, but also human and animal life would be unimaginable. Hence, without water there would be no life. Water is one of the three necessities of life: *water*, *air* and *food* — three absolute essentials that are so much taken for granted. The most obvious uses of water are for drinking, for cooking and for our personal hygiene. Rarely do we stop to think that in today's industrialised society water has become an expensive commodity. The use of water has increased so much that, while the water reserves on this planet remain constant, we are in danger of reaching the stage when the demand for water cannot be met.

Water is of vital importance to our health. Not only is it a medicine for people who are sick, but it is also important that those who are healthy drink at least 1 litre of liquid a day, and better still, 2 litres each day. What is of equal importance in our modern society is that the water we drink is of an acceptable quality. Our very existence depends on the quality of our environment, and the latter, unfortunately, is under constant threat from adverse atmospheric influences. It is sad to reflect on mankind's negligence in its regard for the three sources of energy: *water*, *air* and *food*.

* We frequently hear about food contamination, such as bacterial infections etc., through the media. Just

think of the recurring reports on salmonella outbreaks, especially the salmonella-infected eggs scare in 1989. We have also lived through the panic surrounding the possible link between soft cheeses and listeria.

* The dangers of air pollution also receive considerable publicity through the reporting of damage to the ozone layer caused by excessive exhaust gases and the use of CFC gases in aerosol sprays and refrigerators.

* The facts of water pollution, however, are often side-stepped or overlooked and it is specifically these issues I want to deal with in this book.

Yet the scope of this book goes beyond the issues concerning the pollution of our water supplies, important though these are; I wish to discuss *all* aspects of water, including its positive remedial and therapeutic properties and how we can exploit water as a natural resource for improving our health.

While I was still quite young I was fortunate to be taught about some of the functions that water can perform in natural healing practices by my grandmother, who was a dedicated advocate of the Kneipp methods. Water is a natural medicine that is important for the whole body and should represent a part of our daily routine in the interests of our health. Without water our reserves of energy would quickly and drastically diminish. We have all experienced at some time or other, when we are feeling tired or a bit listless, how a long drink of cold water can give us just that little lift we need. Also, if we take a bath at the end of a hard day, we will feel reinvigorated; equally, at the start of a new day, taking a shower or bath will make us feel bright and alert, ready to tackle whatever lies ahead.

It appears to me that often we fail to recognise the value of this wonderful commodity. The free availability of water in our Western society has become such a routine expectation that it is very much taken for granted.

However, I would like to think that I am not alone in wondering about what has been happening to our water and how badly mankind has interfered with this gift from nature. The Water Act of 1989 has now come into force with its many regulations, some of which will undoubtedly affect the consumer. The standards that have been set by the World Health Organisation (see page 52) are most important, yet the threat of pollution remains with us at all times. The source of water may differ from one country to another and even from one area to another within any given country. Yet even rainwater that is filtered through chalk and therefore comparatively free from pollution is still subsequently interfered with through chemical additives that impair its purity.

Surely we must all agree with the statement that without good health it is hard to enjoy life to the full. Indeed, fortunes are made from our desire to achieve optimum health and fitness. Our body comprises such a great deal of water that we cannot deny the fact that we indeed resemble a mobile quantity of water:

* 70% of the weight of our brain is water;
* 75% of our muscles;
* 83% of our kidneys;
* 22% of our bones; and
* 72% of our blood consists of water.

Moreover, water plays a very important role in the vital functions of the body, e.g. digestion, circulation, lubrication, elimination, absorption and regulation. It will therefore be clear why it is so important that the quality of our water should be up to a desirable standard.

We have all heard the saying 'You are what you eat'. The other day I was driving behind an enormous truck which displayed the message 'You are what you drink!'. Nowadays, this concept is less far-fetched than ever before, because it has become clear that impaired water can easily induce health problems. Not all water is of equal quality; we know that because of differences in its taste and smell, and most of us have a preference or dislike for tap water in specific areas of the country. Other differences in water quality, however, cannot be spotted by sight, taste or smell. We need to be able to trust that when we turn on the tap the water that comes gushing out will not endanger our health. Remember that our body constitutes an intricate system of arteries and blood vessels and that our health depends on an efficient circulatory system. We know that 92 per cent of our blood — the river of our life — is made up of water, and it is the water in the blood that carries nourishment to the cells throughout the body and transports toxins away from the cells for elimination. The right quality of water can enable the blood to perform the vital tasks it is expected to do.

To maintain good health we require good water, good food and good air and ensuring their supply is the simplest do-it-yourself method for maintaining good health. In the case of water, therefore, ensuring its quality merits a great deal of care and attention. In many areas of our daily life we have a free choice. We can choose to make alterations to our home, or change our car, or we can select our favourite food. However, to put it in a nutshell, we are unable to choose the water that is piped into our homes. The Department of Health won a major battle some years ago when a law was passed requiring that all packaging of cigarettes carry the warning that smoking can damage our health, and yet the British water authorities are not obliged to issue similar warnings even though in many areas of the country doing so would not be out of place.

Pure water is a versatile component of all natural healing methods. In this context it is interesting to point out that there are at least five areas in the world where it is not unusual for people's natural life-span to extend beyond one hundred years, in good health. The local inhabitants of these areas will tell you that it is their water that holds the secret of their prolonged life. Whether this is true or not, it is nevertheless interesting to note that in these areas, such as Tibet, Mongolia, Ecuador and Peru, the water is rich in natural colloids and organic poly-electrolytes. The discovery of colloidal structures in the water in Hunza Land, where the locals are renowned for their longevity, has also been greeted with excitement by scientists.

The World Health Organisation advises that we drink a minimum of eight glasses of water every day. This is indeed sound advice, but let us make sure that the water we drink is of a quality that is not substandard. Both the quantity and the quality of our drinking water are vital in the determination of a healthy life. To ensure that the supply of our drinking water is fit for consumption by our children and further generations to come, drastic measures will be required to protect our environment. To safeguard ourselves for the future we have to ensure that our drinking water is kept as natural as possible.

In my book *Viruses, Allergies and the Immune System*, I wrote about an elderly farmer and his wife who were undoubtedly the victims of allergic reactions to substandard water, which in this case had been contaminated by pesticides and other chemicals. The effects were seen clearly in the farmer, who was affected by Parkinson's disease, while his wife had fallen victim to the virus myalgic encephalomyelitis (also known as ME or post-viral syndrome). It is generally difficult to establish conclusively whether the water authorities are guilty of establishing or condoning chemical pollution and we must therefore stay alert at all times. If it is true that Alzheimer's disease, as is feared, is yet another water-borne health problem, is it possible that the aluminium content in the water has any bearing? Many a time when I see a patient who suffers from persistent problems, I wonder to what extent these can be ascribed to toxicity of the water.

Certainly, many rural areas are still serviced by lead water pipes. Yet in the Scottish Highlands, for example, there still exist sources of crystal clear water. I have been given a little device, issued by the Highland Spring Water distributors, which tells us exactly in which areas we find high contents of aluminium, lead, nitrates, pesticides, triahlomethanes etc. in the water. Please let us refrain from unnecessary interference with our water, and try instead to keep it unspoilt.

It must be reassuring to know that, as a rule, we may consider our tap water safe to drink and that it poses minimal health risks. Yet let us never make the assumption that tap water is, and will remain, *completely safe* for consumption, even if we invest in filters for our domestic use. We owe it to our families and to society in general to accept our responsibility to take an active interest in ensuring that the water from our taps will remain safe to use. Investigative research remains necessary and I hope that in some ways this book can help the reader to realise what can be done with nature's wonderful gift for the benefit of mankind — H_2O.

2

Water from the Tap

HOW CAN WE BE SURE that tap water will not endanger our health? It is very important that we know what has happened to the water we drink. On several occasions I have turned on the tap and brown water has trickled out. When I subsequently telephoned the water authorities they would respond: 'Well, it may be difficult, but we'll see what can be done about it.' Then, a few days later, the appearance of the water from the tap would change from brown to a milky opaque liquid. Still more chemicals must have been added to try and purify the existing supply of water. Is this the right answer or are we merely spoiling the water supply further by adding even more chemicals?

Does the Water Act of 1989 truly supply us with the assurance we seek that the water being discharged from our taps can be considered safe with regard to our health? Certainly, I don't doubt that the water authorities are doing their best; nevertheless, we should not shrink from the task of making them responsible to the general public because, after all, we are the consumers and as such we have the right to expect the authorities to act in our best interests.

A perfect example of the far-reaching effects ordinary tap water can have on our health can be experienced by many of us if we spend our holidays in a foreign country. Many tourists suffer from constipation during their holidays, for which the change of water is often blamed. More tourists, however, especially if visiting southern countries with a hot climate, experience the opposite to this complaint, i.e. loose bowels or diarrhoea — again blamed on the drinking water. With an often superior attitude we then claim that the water supply in those holiday resorts is of a substandard quality. Let me tell you of the time I was involved in a practice in Birmingham in the Midlands, an area that has seen a recent influx of Asian immigrants. Countless newly arrived Asians fell ill during their first weeks in this country and attended the clinic with problems such as colitis, diarrhoea, stomach cramps, skin irritations and headaches. It did not take me long to discover that most of these complaints were the result of the change in the drinking water, and when the patients followed my instructions to use only bottled water, their problems were soon solved.

Only a short while ago, at my practice in Lancashire, I saw quite a few patients who had suddenly become ill, suffering from 'flu-like symptoms coupled with a rise in body temperature, while a large percentage also reported skin irritations. Eventually, it became known that the local tap water had been contaminated and a large number of the local population were suffering some rather unpleasant side-effects as a result. This experience provides yet another example of why interference with this valuable commodity should not be tolerated.

Public concern for the safety and quality of our public water supply will bring great pressure to bear on the newly privatised water authorities. Supporters of privatisation believe that the local authorities will continue to remain responsible for maintaining adequate safety standards and that their responsibility will change insofar as they will now perform the role of 'watchdog' to ensure that stringent standards of hygiene and non-impairment are maintained. It is important that the public remain entitled to exert pressure in relation to decisions concerning the chemical additives and other procedures that are supposedly meant to enhance the quality of our water supplies. Never forget that the water authorities must be ultimately accountable to us — the consumers.

Do not hesitate to contact your local water authority if you think that the plumbing in or into your home may be less than adequate. There are still many older properties where the plumbing system or water supply system contains lead pipes.

You should also make sure that when you turn on the tap first thing in the morning you always let the water run for a few minutes so that the supply pipes can be cleared of water that has been standing overnight. Never fill the kettle from the hot-water tap because that water will have been heated the previous night and then allowed to cool down before being heated again. The mineral content will therefore have diminished and will diminish yet further when it is brought to the boil in the kettle. Always empty the kettle after use and when boiling water is next required refill the kettle with water from the cold tap. If you are in any doubt about the standard of the water piped into your home, do not hesitate to seek the advice of an environmental health officer.

I was recently given a brochure published by one of the water authorities, which made very interesting reading. In the introduction it acknowledges that the various reports on environmental water pollution and the quality of tap water often appear controversial. Growing public awareness of environmental pollution has made the consumer more alert and critical — and understandably so, considering the important role water plays in our lives. After all, we all use water, we all need water and so it

My Story

Darren Bailie

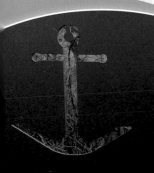

Welcome to
Portavogie

My name is Darren Bailie. My twin brother, Lawson, and I were born in the fishing village of Portavogie on 16th August 1973. Both of us were born with severe physical disabilities, including profound deafness. To make matters worse, after we were born our mum became seriously ill. Consequently, auntie Jean and uncle Hugh stepped in to help, giving me the blessing of a Christian home.

My schoolteacher, Miss Beck, and my Sunday School teacher, Mr Henry Wills, told me Bible stories and taught me from the Word of God. Therefore, from my earliest years I knew right from wrong. I was able to do well at school and gained the Child Achievement Award in London.

After school, I was employed by the NHS and learned to drive. This gave me some independence. Sadly, I started going to gamble at the bookies most Saturdays. Although my family disapproved of this, they were praying for me. Auntie Jean said I was good at betting, but at the same time, she didn't like that sort of money coming into her house.

On my 30th birthday I was given a Bible, which I kept at my bedside. From time to time, I would read it.

I knew about Heaven and Hell since my Sunday school days, but I still asked auntie Jean questions about these.

Around 2007 I began reading Gospel tracts and started attending church more often. I attended a baptism service and this led me to ask my Auntie Jean how I could get to Heaven. She told me I needed to be saved and ask the Lord Jesus into my heart so that I could, one day, be in Heaven.

It was on 18th Jan 2008 that I trusted Jesus Christ as my Saviour. When Auntie Jean asked me how I knew I was saved, I pointed her to John 3:16;

"For God so loved the world, that he gave his only begotten Son, that whosoever believeth in him should not perish, but have everlasting life."

I indicated "**the world**" included me. She further asked if I believed this to be true. I answered her affirmatively with great assurance.

My life was greatly changed. I no longer wasted money at the bookies. Even when my brother Lawson gave me the newspaper to see the runners (horse racing) I told him I was now saved and was no longer interested in gambling. I also started to pray for Lawson and gave him Gospel tracts.

As a Christian I started to attend Portavogie Free Presbyterian Church. It was a great help to me when the minister, Rev. Armstrong, printed his sermons as I could not hear. Despite my physical difficulties, the Lord gave me opportunities to share my testimony. My auntie Daphne greatly helped me with this.

Although I am a Christian I am not exempt from trials. It was a very difficult time when my mum passed away and two years later, my older brother also passed away. I had a difficult time in work, but again the Lord promised in 1 Peter 5:7;

> **"Casting all your care upon Him, for He cares for you."**

I have really proved this to be true.

All my family was present when I was baptised on 27th February 2010 at the Radisson Hotel. It was great to witness to them.

I now live for the Lord. Although I cannot speak, I can pray for those who are not saved. I also witness for Him by sending text messages to family and friends who need the Lord Jesus.

Hebrews 6:19

> **"Which hope we have as an anchor of the soul, both sure and stedfast..."**

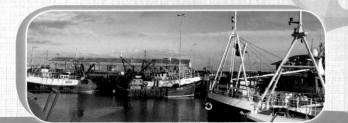

stands to reason that we all want to know what procedures are followed to improve and/or maintain the quality of water so that it is fit for human consumption. So, what happens to water in the purification process?

Technical explanations often act as an 'overkill' as they mostly result in more queries than answers. Statistics on the quality of our tap water may be studied, but rarely do these figures explain the lengthy process required to safeguard our water supplies. Who is involved in this process? How is the water treated? Who is responsible for a plentiful supply? The brochure set out to answer some of these questions.

—The *engineer's* task is to ensure that the consumer can at all times expect a supply of running water when the tap is turned on. Many years ago water was pumped manually, but electronic technology has revolutionised the water industry. Computerisation has changed the function of the water board engineer to a supervisory capacity. This modern equipment is programmed to select the pump capacity according to demand.

—One of the tasks of the *hydrologist* is to produce a long-term forecast of water requirements. Short-term predictions will also be taken into account, such as days when there may be excessive demand or unusually low demand. New Year's Day is an excellent example of the latter, because there are very few families who will decide to use the washing machine on this date.

When the construction of a new housing estate is being considered, the hydrologist is involved with the town planners from the very early stages in the planning procedure to ensure that the water supply will be adequate.

—The *analyst* has the responsibility for ensuring that the water supply complies with the prescribed safety guidelines; for example, if the legal safety limit for a certain

19

substance has been set at 100 micrograms per litre, the water authorities are likely to impose a maximum level of 30 micrograms on their output. Sporadically the concentration of this substance in the water output may increase to 40 or even 50 micrograms per litre, in which case the analyst will ensure that all efforts will be taken to reverse this situation. It is his aim to remain well within the legal limits.

The 'acid rain' syndrome is used as an example in this context. Apparently, the aluminium content in the water has slightly increased as a result of acid rain. In co-operation with certain research authorities, an experimental filter has been developed by this particular authority and the early indications are that it appears to be effective. It is intended that the filter will be applied before too long in the pump installation.

—The *district manager*, although he may have a technical and engineering background, has a mainly administrative function. He forms the link between the water authority and the local authorities. In his line of duty he attends meetings with developers and council representatives. If, for example, road facilities are to be upgraded or street repairs are planned, the water authorities will use this opportunity to check the condition of the water mains while the road repairs or construction are being undertaken. Where possible, the mains will be placed under the pavements instead of under tarmacadam surfaces. The cause of a drop in water pressure in any given area may be damage to the mains, which often used to be located under the tarmacadam surface in the centre of the road. This would not only be difficult to discover, but also costly to repair. Moreover, the increasing weight of traffic can cause water mains to fracture, whether it be due to a gradual shift in the soil or to an increase in the permitted weight of heavy goods vehicles. As a precautionary measure, therefore, many water boards have now changed their practices and prefer to site the mains under the pavements.

— Last but not least, the task of the *repairs officer* is considered in the brochure. In an interview with a repair man we read about the urgency with which defects must be made good. Such emergency call-outs constitute only part of a job in which maintenance is of major importance. At any time the repairs officer may be called away from a routine maintenance job to attend to the repair of a burst or fractured water main — and this, he maintains, adds variety to his job.

Like me, I doubt if many readers ever give a thought to this organisation when they turn on the tap. Quite understandably, most of us take it for granted that a decent quality of drinking water is always available and never give a second thought to the complex organisation responsible for this. Do we ever stop and think about the possibility of the tap water in our region being subject to contamination by substances such as aluminium, lead, nitrates or pesticides? Certainly, if care is taken many contamination problems can be avoided.

I was certainly pleased to learn that the British government is at present coming under pressure from other European governments to adhere to the EEC regulations on water. We are informed that for economic reasons it has not yet been possible to replace all lead pipes with pipes made of a non-toxic substance. An increasing number of reports now point to the disappointing lack of investment in the water industry during recent decades. What has happened to the British promises of ten years ago that we would put our house in order?

It would surprise me if you considered the cost of water to be excessive if you realised that the average person uses 130 litres of water each day — the equivalent of approximately 30 gallons. All that at an average cost of 13 pence per day. It is ironical that two of the three sources of life, i.e. water, air and food, come at such a low price. Should this not give us even greater reason to treasure what we have and to take responsible care of our good fortune?

On the whole bottled water appears a safe option for drinking purposes, but again a word of warning is needed. Some of the sparkling varieties may contain added ingredients to enhance their appeal to the consumer. However, these additives may not always meet the statutory requirements, as was recently the case with Perrier water. Fortunately, this particular product has now been declared completely safe again, but it still leaves one wondering. Carbonated water may appear more palatable, but ask yourself whether your favourite bottled water is naturally carbonated. I dare say that carbonation in itself need not necessarily be detrimental, but it rarely makes the water crisper, cleaner or of better quality. If you are in the habit of using bottled water, make sure that the label states that the water has been tested and approved. Fortunately, the advertising watchdogs are strict in monitoring compliance with their objectives that no claims should be made about a product unless their validity has been proven without doubt.

Always pay attention to the colour and texture of tap water. A hint of cloudiness may be a sign of excessive chlorination. If the water is foaming it may indicate some bacterial contamination and then it will be essential to boil the water before using it. Very often, if the water is contaminated in some way it will have an unusual smell or taste. It should also be noted that if you use a water filter but do not change it frequently enough, this can be a contributor to bacterial growth. Thus if you have decided to use a filter, this does not necessarily mean that you are in the clear. A large variety of filters are obtainable nowadays, ranging from the simple plastic jug variety to extremely sophisticated ones. In a *Which* consumer report published in February 1989 we can read about the results of tests on filtered water. An increase in harmless bacteria was found in samples from jugs which had been left standing for six weeks, even though the activated carbon contained silver. Some filters can become a breeding ground for bacteria and the regular cleaning or replacement of filters is essential.

It appears that the practice of water recycling is becoming increasingly common — worldwide. One might wonder if this is really the answer to our problems, or do we merely initiate other problems through this purification process? So many additives are used in the recycling purification that I am doubtful about the eventual outcome. Water purification in itself is not a new concept. The Sanskrits recorded around the year 2000 BC that it was advisable to purify water before drinking it by boiling it. It was recommended that this be done by dipping a hot copper rod into the vessel containing the supply of drinking water. Also from history we know that the quantity of water used in Imperial Rome was in excess of 200 million gallons a day and that lead conductors were used. Thankfully, nowadays we know about the dangers that lead imposes on our water supplies, even though it is still in use in our present water supply system in Britain.

In 1988 the well-known herbalist Kitty Campion and I did a study on water. We presented our findings in an article entitled 'Water — as lethal as a chemistry set', the contents of which are reproduced below.

> Large numbers of water treatment plants both in Britain and in the United States of America simply do not meet with either Federal or EEC standards. Besides which our environment is now so polluted that water treatments simply do not work adequately to filter these out. In 1978 a paper by the General Accounting Office of the United States said that 'the nation's water supplies are threatened by the careless use of hundreds of chemical compounds and the heedless disposal of toxic waste'. More than 600 of these contaminants have been found in drinking water, half of them proven poisons, fifty-five of them pesticides. By 1990 there will be more than 70,000 such chemicals in use.

Early in 1987 the Department of the Environment published a report admitting an overall deterioration in the health of British rivers since 1980. This is worst in the North-West and South-West of England but increasingly serious in the Midlands. Its findings make a nonsense of the expressed aim of water authorities, which pollute rivers with sewage and monitor the effects. Every step forward is now coupled with two steps back. When the water authorities were established in 1974 their main task was to achieve a massive cleaning of the country's rivers and estuaries by the early 1980s.

The report blames the poor showing on two main factors: dilapidated and overloaded sewage works that can no longer purify sewage adequately before pouring it into rivers, and farm run-offs such as silage and slurry. This must be coupled with the fact that investment by the water authorities in sewers and sewage works has, for the past five years, been half the amount reached in the mid 1970s. It is not fair to simply blame the regional water authorities. The entire industry is underfunded by £100 million a year, and over recent years has been badgered into arbitrary and damaging external financing limits in order not to increase the Public Sector Borrowing Requirement. Such criticism should be aimed at those who set the investment limits: the government.

The Nitrate Scandal
Britain is about to be sued by the EEC because of the illegal levels of nitrates which come mainly from artificial fertilisers in drinking water. The EEC drinking water directive issued in 1985 clearly stated that no drinking water should contain more than 50 mg per litre of nitrate at any one time. The British government chose to interpret the directive differently, by allowing supplies to exceed that level at times, as long as the *average* pollution over a three-month stretch stayed beneath it. They also decided to relax the standard 80 mg per litre simply because their medical advisers cannot currently detect a health risk from nitrate levels up to 100 mg per litre. By relaxing standards for nitrates, the Department of the Environment has postponed having to spend an estimated £200 million. Even after this manoeuvre, the government had to admit that fifty-two water supplies still exceed its limits.

On Mothering Sunday

Delight yourself
in the Lord,
and He will give you
the desires of your heart.

Psalm 37:4

Areas affected include Lincolnshire, Norfolk, Staffordshire, Yorkshire and areas supplied by Anglian and Severn Trent Water Authority. Because of the accelerating nature of a problem caused by nitrate-based fertilisers on dry, arable lands and contamination, it is sure to get worse. Britain admits that 921,000 people receive more than 50 mg per litre over three months, but actually five million people receive water that exceeds the true EEC standards, going over the limit sometimes. Britain has applied for the fifty-two supplies to be exempted from the EEC rules but the Commission, happily, is unlikely to accept this.

The Effects of Nitrates
In the alimentary tract ingested nitrate can break down to nitrite, which is a known toxic factor, and in some cases when a person has no neutral hydrochloric acid in the stomach it can break down even further to nitrosamines, which are known to be potentially carcinogenic and when experimentally used in rats have produced cancers of the bladder, kidneys, nasal sinus, lungs, bronchii, oesophagus, stomach, intestines, nervous system and skin. Ingested nitrate destroys vitamins A and E and may give rise to mineral imbalances and hormone disturbances. In 1937 a study in which 36 mg of nitrate was given to men resulted in decreased blood pressure and circulatory collapse. Studies in East Anglia and Yorkshire involving more than thirty rural areas have found that districts with high nitrate levels also had higher than average instances of stomach cancer, though no causal links were found. However, there is little doubt that nitrates cause methaemaglobinaemia in bottle-fed babies, where the infant effectively suffocates because the blood cannot obtain sufficient supplies of oxygen. The last recorded case in this country was in 1972.

Solutions to Water Pollution
The most obvious solution is to shut off the industrial pollutants at source. Industrialists try their best to scare us off with the fact that filtering out all pollutants would mean higher prices, but many would not mind paying a little more for a really good product, especially if we knew it was actively helping to keep our environment clean and not

endangering health, however marginally. If there is a risk that others are not willing to pay the price, the ethical response from the industrialist is to decide whether the possible reward is worth the risk.

It seems grossly unfair that the polluter — intensive agriculture — is not asked to foot the bill for the mess it spawns. Indeed, the taxpayer ends up paying for mopping up the mess not just once, but three times. Firstly by subsidising intensive agriculture, secondly by paying for the water authorities to remove nitrate pollution and thirdly by footing the bill for the more unquantifiable social costs of the damaging effects on both human health in particular and the environment in general. In order to reduce the nitrates we also need to move to organic farming methods. The fertiliser industries have developed a whole range of new compounds which emulate a biological system by artificially preventing more complex forms of nitrogen developing into nitrates and these compounds are more acceptable environmentally. But it is surely insane to squander millions of pounds and use up large quantities of fossil fuels when crops can be grown naturally in the first place.

There is no doubt that agriculture provides the bulk of free nitrates currently found in the environment. Such nitrates are found in porous rock beneath farmland and are almost impossible to remove. The only solution is to prevent groundwater contamination. The British Geological Survey confirms that changes in farming practice could help. The London Food Commission calls for more research into the development of vegetable crops with low nitrate levels and the adoption of biological growing methods.

All of this is commendable but it may be too little, too late. There is an overwhelming fear among water scientists and environmentalists that we are only just beginning to feel the effects of the huge burden of nitrate pollution. We are literally sitting on a time-bomb. Nearly one-third of our water supplies comes from groundwater, and water can sit in aquifers for more than twenty years before it is used, which means that the water we currently drink could pre-date intensive agriculture. The worst may be yet to come. In the future it could be that we have no choice but to drink bottle or filtered water.

3

Water for Healing

IT CAN HARDLY be an exaggeration to say that water may well be considered the most versatile medicine in existence. Water may be drunk for our health and water may be used for the purposes of medical treatment. Yet it is often overlooked that water is also a component of the air we breathe. When talking of water for healing purposes, consider the benefits to a bronchitic or asthmatic patient who lives near the sea. Think also of those people who suffer from skin conditions. Although Father Sebastian Kneipp (see page 58) had not studied medicine in the accepted sense of the word, he certainly realised that moisture, or dampness, in a concentrated form is beneficial for certain health conditions, and with that thought in mind he introduced certain bath treatments.

Father Kneipp successfully recommended herbal baths for angina, headaches and colds. For rheumatic and arthritic problems he advised foot baths or even full body baths, combining the effects of his steam treatments with those of certain healing herbs. For the latter conditions he also advocated alternate cold and hot water treatments in combination with poultices. On alternate nights either a kaolin poultice or a cabbage leaf is bound over the aching joint, and is left on all night. This is followed in the morning by sluicing hot and cold water over the specific area alternately, or by immersing it in alternate hot and cold baths.

Neuralgic patients usually suffer from a high uric acid content and if they accustom themselves to drinking larger than usual quantities of water they will benefit. People who suffer from painful circulatory afflictions such as varicose veins or haemorrhoids will find relief from the old-fashioned method of placing an ice-cube or ice-cold towels on the affected area. After placing an ice-cube on the haemorrhoid area, it is advisable to take a cold sitz bath and also to have a cold foot bath every night before retiring. Water treatments are also used successfully in the treatment of open wounds, menopausal or menstrual difficulties and prostate problems. Sluicing the appropriate area with cold water or using water poultices will usually bring relief.

The reason for the former popularity of water treatments becomes clear when we consider the communication problems previous generations had to cope with. If there was an illness in the family it was not simply a case of lifting the telephone receiver to call for a doctor or ambulance. Even if the family could afford to pay for the services of a physician, it would often be necessary to set off on foot to fetch the doctor. Moreover, in the depths of winter many households would be totally isolated for long periods and when an illness occurred they would therefore have to be inventive and use whatever knowledge was available to the best of their ability. Such knowledge would often have been handed down by mothers and grandmothers, and in many cases those tried and tested remedies and treatments would be successful; it is to our loss, therefore, that we have allowed them to lapse and make way for more modern treatments. Many natural skills have been lost, but fortunately the wheel is turning full circle and more and more people are now prepared to give natural methods another chance.

Let me give you a word of caution in relation to water treatments. When it is advised to use very hot or very cold water, we are talking about extreme temperatures such as 43 °C (110 °F) for hot water and about –9 °C (15 °F) for cold water. Such extremes are not always suitable if the patient concerned is very young or elderly; hence, use your common sense when deciding whether to opt for a therapy that involves the use of very hot or very cold water. Having said that, I will remind you that as a healer water will stimulate the internal organs and will assist the body to fight off intruders. An internal wash in the form of water taken orally or via the colon is still considered to be one of the quickest ways to rid the body of toxins.

Of course, water for healing needs to be of a good quality and unfortunately this has become a somewhat rare substance, despite the fact that three-quarters of the earth's surface is covered by water.

I cannot remember who coined the phrase that 'the skin is the keyboard of hydrotherapy', but this saying does reveal an enlightened mind. Given the correct natural environment, the skin will perform its task well. The body is able to produce heat in two ways: firstly by oxidation through burning up food such as fats, and secondly by the activity of different parts of the body. Heat is generated while the heart beats and blood is pumped through the body. Heat is also produced in the body as the result of other processes such as metabolic activity, physical exertion and even by the emotions. When heat is produced within the body, we perspire. The blood flows to the surface of the skin, where its temperature is reduced. The blood flowing through the layers of the skin cools down through the skin's contact with the air. As the blood continues to circulate, this process is maintained until a comfortable temperature is obtained.

29

This process never ceases to surprise people when they realise how competently the body functions are programmed. The skin is also an indicator of our state of health. The skin will heal and recover more quickly from a surface injury if it is sponged down with cold water, which accelerates its healing activity and hardens the skin. An overall cold sponging or shower will uplift us; not only does it revitalise our energy level, but in its own way it is beneficial to our nervous system. Try it when you feel depressed and you may be pleasantly surprised.

'Prevention is better than cure' is a valid axiom at any time, but never more so than nowadays when problems such as *Candida albicans*, post-viral syndrome (ME), allergies and viruses are so prevalent. I have also noticed a vast increase in the number of people complaining of digestive problems. Digestion begins in the mouth and its efficiency is highly dependent on the salivary glands. Masticating, or chewing, is not only necessary to break down food into a size that can be easily swallowed; a further important function of this process is the mixing of saliva with the food, which greatly enhances the later stages of digestion. You will understand that the success of this process is also dependent on the quality of water. The soft lining of the stomach contains a number of small glands that produce gastric juices and between them these glands produce between 5 and 10 litres of juice each day. These glands can be easily overworked and their efficiency is by no means enhanced if the quality of our water is substandard. Many stomach problems can be avoided if our drinking water is of good quality.

Sinus problems and neuralgias respond well to the application of heat, and especially if the pains are severe, hot and cold compresses are useful. If you are bothered with severe neuralgia pains when you awake in the morning, run some comfortably hot water over the area and then repeat using cold water and you will find that the discomfort will be much relieved. When suffering from severe hay fever attacks, alternate hot and cold foot baths will relieve the condition considerably, and the same treatment is advisable when suffering from a headache.

As a naturopath I find myself repeatedly stressing the point that the system needs to be detoxified. Although the body is equipped with its own excellent means for detoxification, the overload on the system in most walks of life is considerable. Cleansing the system can be done very successfully by fasting, in which case the quality of drinking water used is of the utmost importance. In order to thoroughly detoxify the body of some of the pollutants that are lurking in our system, an adequate supply of minerals such as calcium, zinc and magnesium is essential. Vitamin C will also be beneficial in helping the body to rid itself of traces of pesticides, chemical additives and other toxic substances. At the best of times it is difficult to eliminate pesticide traces from the system and this function cannot be performed by water alone. Supplements of additional anti-oxidants may then be called for.

In this connection I must tell you about a letter I received from a lady who had recently learned that she suffered from multiple food allergies and had been informed that this condition had been caused by the water she was drinking. After investigation it was discovered that she had an intolerance to chlorine and certain other chemicals that were added to the water. She was advised to invest in a charcoal filter for her tap and before long her problems were overcome. In her letter she proudly informed me that she was now able to eat anything she fancied — something she had not been able to do for a long time. A simple change in the composition of her tap water made that possible for her.

Recently, considerable medical interest has been expressed in hydrotherapy in relation to the treatment of heart disease. During the course of investigations on various naturopathic approaches it was found that some forms of heart disease react very well to certain types of water treatment, and this angle was subsequently examined in greater detail. An increase in blood pressure results in greater activity of the heart. As the heart has to cope with an extra workload, there is a decrease of the hormonal secretion called *atrial natriuretic hormone,* or *ANP.* This hormone is circulated to the kidneys, where excess sodium is removed from the blood. The resultant drop in salt (sodium) levels then produces an automatic excretion of water. Finally, the reduction in the fluid in the body causes the blood pressure to fall. When the patient is otherwise in good health this method can be used very effectively to reduce high blood pressure.

Both Dr Alfred Vogel and I have advocated hydrotherapy for many conditions and we both favour the use of water as a healer, specifically in cases of kidney, gallbladder and liver complaints. I came across an interesting case some time ago in the Netherlands, where a patient's blood pressure had suddenly increased drastically. Initially I was somewhat puzzled because the patient stated categorically that she had not made any changes to her diet that could have resulted in this condition. However, she eventually let slip that she had changed her preference in mineral water. She had taken to drinking 'Spa Red', which contains considerable quantities of sodium. At my instigation she reverted to her former choice, 'Spa Blue', and her blood pressure soon regulated itself.

In 1488 the royal seal of approval was given to water that was fit for human consumption, and His Majesty King James IV of Scotland paid the staggering sum of twelve shillings for a barrel of local ale that had been prepared using water from a famous spa. Most tests on spa waters come to the same conclusion and this water, from the Ochil Hills in Perthshire, is no exception — namely, it has an unusually low sodium content.

In Chapter 7, which deals with water pollutants, I explain in greater detail the harm that can result from excessive levels of chlorine and fluoride in water. These chemicals are added purposely, but what about the other pollutants that enter our water system more or less undetected from sources such as water drawn from agricultural areas where artificial pesticides and fertilisers have been allowed to contaminate the water supply? Or what about water that is recycled over and over again? Previous generations may not have had the advantages of having water piped into their homes through a mains supply, but they were better off from the point of view that their water was obtained direct from spas or wells. It appears that even in those days there existed considerable superstition concerning the use of certain waters. Stories abound about water from specific sources being endowed with certain properties, such as its ability to overcome infertility. Personally, I can hardly believe that. Yet some of my elderly patients would insist on going to the former St Enoch Station in Glasgow if they were bothered with bronchitis or with skin diseases. When you walked underground at this station there would be a constant drip of water from above, and it was claimed that if you allowed the drops to land on the affected parts of the body, certain problems would be cured. I know some people who would even insist on drinking the water for these purposes. It is, of course, possible that this water could have been filtered through a layer of mineral or trace elements, in which case some of the claimed remedial factors can be explained scientifically.

In the above context we may have to settle for accepting the principle that the mind is more powerful than the body. The individual's positive belief that certain water contained specific remedial properties would in itself have had a beneficial effect. In some parts of Scotland it was firmly believed that extraordinary curative properties were to be found in the waters from Scottish running wells. For example, on the first Sunday in May parents would take their sick children, including youngsters who suffered from tuberculosis, to one particular well, where it was claimed the waters contained healing properties. I have never been able

33

to discover what was so special about the specific date, but apparently these curative powers were only available on the first Sunday in May. Stories also exist about a well where people would supposedly find relief from toothache. There were some wells of which it was claimed that any affliction or illness would be cured after taking the waters. Indeed, some remarkable stories have been related on the curative properties of specific sources of water. As early as the year 1260 it was claimed that the waters of the Pannanick Wells would cure people of scorbutic and scrofulous complaints. Then there was the Bridgeheader Well, where apparently the water came from three sources and the water from each individual source was recommended for a specific purpose: blindness, loneliness and deafness. Records tell how yet another well was frequented by people who hoped to protect themselves from catching the plague.

Am I being too cynical when I suggest that all this could only have been based on sheer superstition? However, where well water has been analysed, the results tend to indicate that it contains higher than usual quantities of calcium, magnesium, silver, iron and silica. Therefore I can readily accept that drinking such waters could well benefit one's general health, because such minerals and trace elements would quickly boost the immune system. You may now more readily understand my conviction that water can be a true healer. Let us, however, always make sure that the water used for drinking, for bathing or for any medicinal use is of the highest quality.

How about making a slight alteration to the old adage 'You are what you eat'? I would suggest that there is an equal amount of truth in the version I noted earlier: 'You are what you drink'. Hippocrates, the father of medicine, impressed upon his students: 'Let our food be our medicine'. On the same basis I feel that water should also be regarded as a medicine. It will then become clear why we are obliged to do everything in our power to keep it pure and natural.

4

Water as a Therapy

AT THE BEGINNING of the twentieth century water therapies were already reputed to be beneficial; especially in those days it was fully accepted that with the use of ice-cold water a drastic change to one's health pattern could be effected within a matter of minutes. My grandmother, who was a true follower of Father Kneipp's water treatment methods, practised a treatment which she claimed would promote longevity, happiness and good health free from blood circulatory problems. One of the things she always mentioned was that if one washed the body with cold water, it should always be done from the right bottom towards the left top. One of the well-known methods she adhered to was to start with the right leg, progressing from the foot up towards the groin, and from the inside to the outside. Then repeat this pattern with the left leg, moving up to the groin and from the inside to the outside. Next, wash the right arm, from the hand to the shoulder — always inside to outside — before repeating with the left arm. Proceed next to the groin area, making circular movements, all the time using ice-cold water. Then move up to underneath the armpits, always in circular movements. Move back to the buttocks, going as high as possible, as far as the neck and shoulders. Finally, wash the face and feet, also in circular movements.

Always remember to keep the flannel wet all the time, just so that it does not drip. When you have finished, very softly towel yourself dry, remembering that after such a cold-water treatment one should never towel the body dry with vigorous movements. In fact, it would be much better to cover the bed with a single sheet and then lie on this until the water has been absorbed by the skin and the body has become dry of its own accord.

Another form of water therapy that is especially recommended for the blood circulation is to brush the whole body with ice-cold water. This treatment is guaranteed to provide you with all the energy and stimulation that you will need for the day ahead if it is done first thing in the morning. It may be repeated in the evening. Personally, I like to go outside in the morning, especially when the dew is still on the grass, and walk barefoot through the wet grass. I also like to do this in freshly fallen snow, and follow this up by placing my feet in a basin filled with cold water in which I exercise my feet. I remember when I spent the period over Christmas and New Year in Switzerland one year. My hostess set me the example of running barefoot around the house immediately after the clock had chimed in the New Year. This was supposed to bring good luck for the forthcoming year. I cannot remember whether that was the case for me or not, but I do recall that it was a most invigorating experience and that afterwards my feet and legs tingled with a sensation of well-being.

Yet other versions of water therapy rely on additions to the bath water, such as some sea salt or Epsom salts to a cold bath, or herbs such as lavender, melissa, rosemary, thyme, juniper berries or pine needles to a bath filled with tepid water. If you feel tired during the day, directing a jet of cold water over both wrists will quickly refresh you. If the opportunity presents itself, you might try resting for a while with the forehead covered by a cloth that has been soaked in ice-cold water. Or if the legs feel tired, you can place a cold, wet cloth over the back of the legs. Repeatedly splashing some cold water over the face, including the eyes, is another speedy way of banishing all traces of weariness.

Water dousing, or localised water treatments, result in a tingling feeling all over the body, as they stimulate the blood circulation. This technique is the simplest form of water therapy imaginable and the water jets may be directed at specific parts of the body. People who suffer from asthmatic or bronchial complaints should always use water at a temperature between 30 and 40 °C (86-104 °F) and never continue the treatment for longer than one minute. If cold water is used, do not extend the treatment beyond 1-15 seconds. Sometimes an ice-cold wet towel or poultice can be effective. One of my teachers was once called to a seriously ill patient who was running a very high temperature. When he saw the patient and realised the danger of the situation, he immediately asked for a large towel, which he then drenched in ice-cold water and placed over the naked body of the patient. He then rolled the patient into a blanket and left him wrapped up in this way for about five minutes. The rapid improvement that resulted from this apparently simple treatment was astonishing. I have often witnessed equally effective results when using poultices, especially in circumstances where I feel that mud or clay poultices are called for.

Of course, water can be used in several different ways; the choice of water therapy depends on the kind of health problems we are dealing with and the general fitness of the patient concerned. Locally, we can use hot-water compresses for the chest, throat, shoulders and spine, all of which will bring quick relief. We can also use cold compresses in the form of an ice pack, which will quickly heat up the body. This effect can also be easily achieved by placing a cold, wet cloth on the relevant area, possibly covered with a sheet of plastic, and then placing a dry towel over the top.

It is also possible to sponge the whole body or localised area with ice-cold water to which some alcohol or surgical spirit has been added; in cases of phlebitis, the addition of some *Hamamelis* (witchhazel) tincture to the water will provide excellent results. The use of sitz baths, foot baths or herbal baths will be equally beneficial, as cold sprays and even steam may be used in conjunction with these methods.

There are so many ways in which water can be used for remedial purposes. As we have seen, hot or cold compresses are very important, but never more so than when they are applied in alternation. Alternate hot and cold compresses help to ease pain and discomfort, such as that experienced as a result of rheumatism, bruised ribs and even nerve pains.

When using cold compresses, always apply one first to the forehead and then another to the affected part. This treatment may last from half an hour up to two hours at a time. I have often found that patients who suffer from sciatic pains sense great relief when a hot, damp compress is placed on the painful limb or area. To prepare such a compress use a soft cotton towel folded into three to resemble a small bandage. Immerse this in hot water, then squeeze out the surplus so that it does not drip. Apply some Bioforce PoHo oil to the affected area before covering it with the warm towel, which is left in place until it has totally cooled down. Repeat this procedure twice. Even patients who are in considerable discomfort will experience quick relief.

When treating throat, neck or ear problems, or coughs, it is better to use a very cold compress. Here again, a cotton cloth or towel should be used, folded in three, this time with some cider vinegar sprinkled on it. A cold compress is also recommended for the treatment of bronchitis, asthma and even emphysema, but in these cases hot towels should then be placed on top of the cold compress. If quick relief is sought by such patients they would do well to place a cold compress on the ninth dorsal of the vertebrae and also to use some PoHo oil.

For constipation, flatulence and other bowel problems it is advisable to use compresses drenched in cold water to which some chamomile has been added.

In cases of haemorrhoids, prostate infections or difficulties with urinating, alternate hot and cold compresses are called for, with a few drops of *Hamamelis* tincture added to the water.

A foot compress is of great help for cramp, hard skin or nerve pain. Rub the feet with some cream or Vaseline, soak some long cotton socks in very hot water, then place these on the feet as soon as the temperature is comfortable to the skin.

It is not an old wife's tale that a hot-water bottle provides relief from menstrual pain. However, it must be used sensibly; always remember that if a metal or rubber bottle is used, it must be wrapped in a towel to prevent the skin being scalded.

Sitz baths are beneficial, as is immersing oneself for a brief period in a bathtub filled with cold water. This also affords an opportunity to practise skin-brushing. The use of a shower is strongly advocated too. Jets of water can be directed at a specific part of the body and either hot or cold water can be used for this purpose, according to need. A cold shower is an excellent means of lowering the body temperature or overcoming tiredness, and is also beneficial if the person concerned has a tendency to faint. Hot showers can help to overcome pain, have a calming effect on the central nervous system and alleviate certain skin complaints. People who enjoy taking a shower would be well advised to try to accustom themselves to alternating the temperature. In many cases I would suggest having a nice warm shower, while occasionally reducing the temperature to cold for a few seconds. Alternate warm and cold showers are of great benefit to the vegetative nervous system, which is generally under constant stress nowadays.

The water from a shower may be directed to the feet, the calves, and the stomach; in the latter case, try to point the shower head directly at the point immediately under the navel. Showers can also be easily directed towards areas that are otherwise difficult to reach, such as the anus or vagina, and here too alternate cold and hot showers are advised.

What really happens as a result of water therapy? When cold water is applied to the skin a prickly feeling is experienced, causing a reflex in the veins and capillaries of the skin. The body subsequently reacts to this and it is this reaction that is so important. In the case of cold water, small muscles will narrow the veins. However, depending on the kind of water treatment selected, one can decide whether to narrow or widen the veins. The narrowing of the veins or capillaries is a result of an active contraction or paralysis of the muscles. Widening comes as a result of the relaxation of these muscles. When the veins narrow, the skin grows visibly paler and becomes cooler; when the veins widen, the skin will become more colourful and warmer. So, through stimulation with the aid of cold water there is an active narrowing of the capillaries and the skin will lose colour; alternatively, the skin will become flushed when the veins widen and the circulation improves.

Certain rules have to be observed when practising any form of water therapy. Before you begin, always make sure that the body is warm and, especially if the person concerned is ill and weak, a good body wash or rub down may be used to prepare the body and make it warm and comfortable. For this purpose use a thick towel and gently rinse the skin a number of times using water only; in other words forget about using soap.

People who are ill would be well advised to have a medium-warm bath of about 37-38 °C (98.6-100.4 °F) and if they wish to alternate this with a cold bath, this may be done by immersing themselves in the latter for no longer than thirty seconds to two minutes — definitely no more.

I am a great admirer of Vincenz Priestnitz, who was a well-known lay practitioner in his day and had a marvellous understanding of the reactions of the skin. He was always extremely hesitant to treat anyone whose skin did not react. It was Priestnitz who stated that any illness and disease that is curable can be cured by hydrotherapy. He claimed that the world's best pharmacy was to be found in water from a fresh spring. I would tend to agree with him, but with certain qualifications, as the cause of impurities in the blood or organs cannot be taken away by water alone. Dietary management must also be considered as an important factor, and let us not forget to check that our lifestyle allows for sufficient rest, sleep and exercise. Only if all these factors are harmoniously balanced do we have the foundation for good health.

Today, it is still true that water can work miracles, but common sense is the ultimate requirement. When I treat members of the younger generation I occasionally read signs of incredulity in their faces when I recommend a simple form of water therapy, and this is generally followed by a look of indulgence. They regard me as 'somewhat cranky'. If they would like to believe this, so be it, but nothing is farther from the truth with regard to the methods I propose. Hydrotherapy is indeed a wonderfully natural way of treating people — and yet so very effective. The treatment for acne — which is especially relevant to the younger generation — is to drink two or three glasses of cold water first thing in the morning and some herbal tea several times during the day. Then I suggest the so-called 'warm-water process'. Having cleansed the skin thoroughly, spread on some Bioforce Cream, drench a towel in hot water and place this over the skin, as warm as the skin can

41

take it. Cover this with a dry towel and leave all this in place until the cream has soaked into the skin. Then cleanse the skin with cleansing milk. If required, this process may be repeated twice. I can guarantee that the patient will be pleasantly surprised with the results.

Arthritic patients will obtain great relief from an old French water therapy, in which a bayleaf infusion is added to the water. Take eight tablespoons of crushed bayleaves, one pint (half a litre) of boiling water and the same quantity of cider vinegar. Place the bayleaves in a heat-resistant container and pour over the boiling water. Cover and leave to infuse for about thirty minutes. Add the vinegar and leave to stand for about one hour, then strain and bottle the infusion. If you add one pint (half a litre) of this liquid to your bath water and relax for fifteen or twenty minutes in the bath, your aches and pains will be eased.

All over the world water treatments have been devised and used in some shape or form. In Scotland it was believed that extraordinary curative properties were to be found in wells. The patient would drink the water and also use it for bathing. St Ninian's Well in Prestwick was used by Robert the Bruce and is even said to have cured him of leprosy.

Father Sebastian Kneipp recommended the application of lightning-fast water treatments for only a few seconds on various parts of the body. The water should be at room temperature and definitely not ice-cold, and the body should be as warm as possible. The whole body should be wetted quickly and the skin should not be rubbed dry; instead, press the water gently into the pores with a sponge or damp towel. As soon as you have completed this procedure you should get dressed and take some exercise to restore your body heat. According to Father Kneipp, blood obstructions are the main cause of disease: 'When these obstructions occur in various parts of the body, the blood remains cooped up, neither able to advance nor retreat properly.' The principle behind his recommendations is simple: water temperature affects the circulation, either by increasing or reducing it. This is especially important when tissues or organs are congested or inflamed.

In China I came across the following instructions, which were often given to rheumatic and arthritic patients. They would be advised to drink six large tumblers of water in quick succession, as this would render the colon more effective in forming fresh blood. This is made possible by the function of the mucosa folds of the colon, or large intestine, which absorb the nutrients obtained from food and utilise them to manufacture fresh blood. The adult colon can be as long as 2.5 metres and is capable of absorbing these nutrients several times a day. For this process to work efficiently, the colonic tract must be clean and receive sufficient exercise; if this is not the case, then the person will feel exhausted and become sick. The blood thus manufactured is responsible for curing our ailments and is considered as a prime power in the improvement of our health. Thus, the water therapy that restores and promotes the body's ability to produce it will make us healthy and prolong our lives.

A sick person may find it difficult to drink large quantities of water, but should persevere nevertheless. Wherever possible, try to take some exercise after drinking the required amount of water. Bedridden people who are unable to get up and do some exercises after having drunk the water should practise deep inspiration and expiration while lying in bed, and massage their stomachs in order to promote the flow of water inside the colon, which will serve to wash and cleanse the mucosa folds. Some people will experience loose bowels and may also have to pass water as often as three times in one hour. However, by using this water treatment, people who are suffering from gastritis may expect to be cured within one week.

Older people who suffer from arthritis or rheumatism should undergo water therapy at least three times a week. They would also benefit if they accustomed themselves to drinking the juice of a raw potato every morning as well as a good quantity of water. Wash a medium-to-large potato, but do not remove the skin. Extract the juice from the potato using a grater. Only a small amount of liquid will be obtained, but this should be diluted with a full glass of water and drunk first thing in the morning. With regular use you will find that the pain will subside.

The old adage 'Prevention is better than cure' still holds true. Many forms of hydrotherapy practised over an extended period will be beneficial to one's general health. Take any opportunity you have to paddle barefoot in the sea or to wade through the running water of a spring. Make it part of your regular routine to have a lukewarm bath and, while relaxing in it, do some breathing exercises.

People with high blood pressure should develop the routine of drinking two glasses of distilled water first thing in the morning. This is an excellent natural way to bring about a reduction in the blood pressure.

To improve the blood circulation my favourite treatment is the 'cold dip'. This exercise should be done each morning on awakening and each night before retiring. Place a basin of cold water at the side of the bed and keep a towel ready. Before rising in the morning place both feet in the water. After counting to ten remove the feet and place them on the towel. Exercise the toes as if you were trying to pick up a marble, doing this 10-30 times. Before going to bed at night follow the same procedure. You will find that your feet are lovely and warm when you snuggle down in bed. The important thing to remember about this exercise is that it should be done for a minimum of sixty sessions to obtain the full benefit. As with some of the other water therapies I have mentioned, do not be fooled into thinking that this procedure is too simple to be effective, because I can assure you that you will experience its considerable benefits if you keep up the routine.

Congestion can be a serious problem and yet this too can be helped by hydrotherapy, applied in the form of showers, compresses or hot and cold foot baths. Again, the routine must be followed over an extended period, but the effects will eventually be noticed.

Bed sores may take a very long time to heal, and here again cold compresses on the affected parts will improve the circulation and so stimulate the healing process.

Headaches are greatly relieved by placing an ice-cold cloth over the occiput and on the forehead. Many people who have tried this have expressed their surprise at the tremendous relief obtained from this simple action.

I am doubtful if a more effective treatment has been devised for tonsillitis and throat problems than the old-fashioned advice Dr Andrew Gold used to give his patients. Dr Gold founded a small hydro in Musselburgh, near Edinburgh, and advocated many forms of cold-water treatment. For tonsillitis and recurring throat problems he advised his patients to fast for seventeen days and to take a cold sitz bath daily. He would also sometimes recommend that a cloth dampened with cider vinegar be wrapped around the neck, or even that cider vinegar be used as a gargle.

For the localised treatment of limbs or joints, such as bruising of knees, elbows, wrists or hands, an ice pack is recommended, or the use of alternate hot and cold compresses or immersions.

Menstrual pains will respond well to water therapy. A week before menstruation is due to take place, take a hot sitz bath on alternate days, and stir some French mustard into the bath water. If the menstrual pains are very painful, you might want to add some chamomile or peppermint to the sitz bath instead. In addition, drink two glasses of cold water every day. Compresses applied to the vertebrae and/or over the stomach will also be helpful. This advice is also useful for people with a nervous disposition.

Most of you will already know this, but I would like to stress here how important it is for people with kidney disturbances that they drink ample quantities of water. In many cases I have noticed that patients prefer to use bottled water for this purpose. By ensuring that they drink plenty, the person concerned may successfully reduce the frequency of some of the painful attacks they have to endure.

Psoriasis is a difficult problem to cure by any means, and yet even here water treatment can be most helpful. In my book *Arthritis, Rheumatism and Psoriasis* I have devoted more time to this problem, but let me remind you here that a person with psoriasis would be well advised never to use soap. Instead, psoriasis patients would be wise to look into such alternatives as salt baths or mud baths. I have seen marvellous results when people have used the mineral salts obtained from the Dead Sea, and many psoriasis clinics advocate the use of these salts. Warm mud compresses have also been found useful, as has sea water. Using these methods improvement can be achieved by people who suffer from this unpleasant condition.

Sinus problems and headaches that occur as a result of sinus conditions will be helped by water baths and steam baths. The addition of a few drops of PoHo oil will enhance the effects of these treatments.

If you experience urinary problems, such as prostate complaints or any other condition that makes the passing of water painful or difficult, try adding some *Solidago* (golden rod) or rosehip to a nice warm bath. After soaking in the bath for about ten minutes, use an enema that has been prepared beforehand using approximately one litre of water to which a dessertspoon of salt has been added. You will soon experience the benefits of this simple treatment.

Some of my patients have appreciatively labelled me as the 'bicarbonate of soda doctor', because I often advise that a handful of bicarbonate of soda is dissolved in the bath water to provide relief from muscular aches and strains.

An excellent home remedy for trauma is to place the feet of the affected person in a bowl of warm water for about five minutes, after which they should be wrapped in a pre-warmed towel. Then gently rub some St John's wort oil into the feet. If on-the-spot treatment is required for a heart patient who has undergone a traumatic experience, it will be helpful to place an ice pack on the left side of the chest over the heart. This should be left in place for a few minutes and then replaced by a warm compress for fifteen seconds. Finally, some PoHo oil should be smoothed onto the chest area. This whole procedure may be repeated twice.

Unfortunately, our modern civilisation has moved on from what were once acceptable and effective treatment methods based on simple requirements that are supplied by nature. This does not mean, however, that such treatments have therefore become ineffective. Consider how instinctively animals react; we all know that if they injure a limb, they will lick their wounds. In this way they will cleanse the wound, but also the rasping quality of the tongue will stimulate the healing process. Cattle will seize any opportunity to wander through muddy or wet patches in the fields; in other words they will treat themselves to a foot bath. Our forebears had that same instinctive knowledge and developed it further by devising various types of water treatment. From history we know that in the Egyptian and Roman civilisations water was held to be of tremendous importance, and not just in the sense of its being a liquid for drinking and for hygienic purposes. They were instinctively aware of its remedial properties and took full advantage of these. Hippocrates, the father of medicine, praised the value of water as a therapy many centuries ago. Today, it is still undoubtedly true that water will therapeutically affect the body, skin and tissues.

5

Water for Cleansing

MORE THAN ONCE I have seen or heard water referred to as a 'liquid of nature', but unfortunately nowadays I often wonder if this synonym remains valid. Our water is interfered with to such a large extent through various circumstances that we have to wonder how natural the water supply is that comes pouring out of our taps. For a variety of environmental and ecological reasons it is now not only required but in most cases essential that our water is subjected to a purification process before it can be used for domestic consumption. This is, in part, the price we have to pay for industrialisation and technical progress. With 'green issues' very much in the news these days, I listened with astonishment to a recent radio broadcast from which I learned that no less than one-third of the water intended for domestic use in France does not undergo any purification measures. Having heard that, I was therefore less surprised to learn that more than one million residents in France are obliged to boil the water from their taps before it is considered relatively safe to use.

I was wondering how to approach this chapter when the answer came to me by way of an encouraging letter I received. The lady who wrote the letter described her experience as follows:

'I have suffered from multiple food allergies for a number of years. These are controlled by rotating my diet.

'Obviously I have an intolerance to chlorine and chemicals which are added to the water. Before I had a charcoal filter fitted to my water supply, it was quite time-consuming for my husband to go to the local farm spring to collect gallons of water in containers (this was checked periodically by environmental health inspectors).

'The filter has made life much easier as I now only have to turn on my tap, knowing it is quite safe to consume the water. I really think this is a great filter and would make life easier for a lot of people. If you would like to ask any questions I would be only too willing to discuss some of the benefits with you. . . .'

A wide range of water filters is being marketed at present, with individual models varying greatly in their complexity, effectiveness and cost. If you decide to take this road, it is extremely important to do your groundwork before selecting the most appropriate type of filter for your needs. If the one I use at home is anything to go by, I can tell you that I consider it essential that it is cleaned on a monthly basis. It never fails to surprise me how many impurities and irregularities are to be found in the filter, and I shudder to think where these would otherwise have ended up and what damage my family may have suffered. However, filtering these visible impurities is only a small part of its function. My basic interest when I decided to use a water filter was in filtering out the unseen chemicals and additives present in the water. The fact that they cannot be seen does not mean they are not harmful.

I recently read in an interesting article some distressing statistics. It is calculated that somewhere in the world, and of course this usually happens in underdeveloped countries, every hour an infant life is lost as a result of diarrhoeal disease spread by dirty water. Over a period of twelve months this gives a total of approximately five million children's lives lost, primarily in the under-five age group. As every parent knows, any illness in a very young child is potentially serious, as the child's condition can deteriorate alarmingly fast. In the hot, dry conditions of some African and Asian regions, dehydration is more than serious — it is a matter of life and death. Once diarrhoeal disease has set in, a baby can die within just two or three days, so one can hardly be accused of exaggeration if it is stated that every minute counts. I am delighted that action groups in Britain have taken it upon themselves to effect a change in these painful statistics with the help of a remedy that has been developed called ORT — Oral Rehydration Therapy. This is one of the simplest and cheapest natural remedies known to science. One full course of treatment costs as little as five pence, and can save a life. A spoonful of sugar and a pinch of salt dissolved in a litre of water is all it takes and ORT takes only twenty-four hours to work — replacing the vital body fluids and salts that are lost when diarrhoea strikes. If you would like to know more about this treatment, or would like to support the charity set up to promote it, please write to:

CARE Britain
36 Southampton Street
London
WC2E 7HE.

The letter I quoted earlier from the lady who wrote to me about her charcoal filter brought back memories of my grandmother, who also used charcoal for water purification. Because of these childhood memories I had already developed an interest in filtration and purification processes and therefore was familiar with the system praised by this lady. My long-standing interest in this subject also served me well in my conversations with a certain chemist who has become a specialist in bone charcoal filtration systems. A Scottish subsidiary of a worldwide conglomerate, considered the world's largest and most technically advanced manufacturer of bone charcoal, has developed a product called BRIMAC 216 Bone Charcoal, which is at the heart of many filtration purification systems in use all over the world.

This bone charcoal has been specifically developed for use in water purification systems for municipal, industrial and domestic applications. It differs from other forms of charcoal and activated carbons in that it contains two separate components — a carbon surface and a hydroxy-apatite lattice — both of which are porous and readily available for adsorption. It is a safe and well-established adsorbent and is used in the sugar-refining industry, other food processes and in aquaculture systems. The use of this bone charcoal in a water treatment system is an efficient and economical method of ensuring that drinking water meets the standards of the EEC directive on water quality. It reduces the levels of toxic or harmful metals such as lead, cadmium, mercury, copper, iron, aluminium, manganese, strontium, arsenic and zinc from water supplies. It also reduces the levels of fluoride, chlorine and certain organic compounds and removes colour, taste and odour from any water supply.

BRIMAC 216 enables the water authorities to ensure that their water output meets the stringent standards agreed with our European partners on water quality. In many instances, charcoal filters can be economically installed — even in remote stations where virtually no chemical treatment exists. The product can be utilised both in slow sand filter systems or in rapid gravity filters. In some cases it can be applied as the principal treatment, while in others

51

it can be used as a final polish prior to disinfection. Its unique buffering properties allow the pH correction of water to be done either without the addition of lime etc. or with a much reduced addition of such alkaline chemicals.

The treatment of private water supplies has become an increasingly important factor in water treatment. In Britain, local environmental health officers are now paying much more attention to the quality of private water supplies. Particularly those industries involved in processing or preparing food are becoming more aware of the need for better water quality. Indeed, the EEC directive on water quality places the responsibility on the end user for the quality of water at the point of entry, even when the water source is that of a municipal authority.

The World Health Organisation sponsored a project to investigate the efficiency of various treatment processes in removing low concentrations of toxic metals in water. The extent of removal of lead, cadmium, inorganic mercury and methyl mercury in coagulation, softening, and by adsorption, were all investigated under laboratory conditions.

International standards set by the World Health Organisation for drinking water give the maximum allowable concentration for lead as 0.10 mg per litre, for cadmium 0.010 mg per litre, and for mercury 0.0010 mg per litre. These metals were added to samples of hard water and soft water (deionised water) to give a concentration that was double the standards laid down by the World Health Organisation.

Coagulation experiments with both aluminium sulphate and ferrous sulphate, at pH values ranging from 6.5 to 8.5, showed that at the 95 per cent turbidity removal dose, lead was removed to below the required standard at each pH value and that lower concentrations were achieved in hard water. Cadmium was only removed to below the set standards at higher pH values, and lower concentrations were not consistently achieved in hard water, as was the case with lead. None of the conditions gave residual mercury concentrations below the World Health Organisation standard.

After softening with calcium hydroxide and using 20 mg per litre ferrous sulphate as a coagulant, samples of hard water and Thames river water showed residual concentrations of lead and cadmium to be less than half the prescribed standard. Some removal of mercury was achieved but in only one case, that of inorganic mercury in river water, was the mercury removed to below the standard considered acceptable.

A study of the adsorption of lead and cadmium from hard and soft water onto two carbons, and onto bone charcoal filters, illustrated that adsorption onto either of the two carbons was far less than that onto the bone charcoal. It has also been shown that the bone charcoal appears to have a high capacity for both organic and inorganic mercury. For all the metals, even better results were obtained in soft water.

As a result of these adsorption experiments, columns were packed with BRIMAC 216 and were fed at different flow rates with water containing lead, cadmium and inorganic mercury. Determination of the lead, cadmium and mercury concentrations of the column effluents showed that removal was dependent on the flow rate. At operating flow rates of the same order as rapid and sand filters, lead could be removed to below the World Health Organisation standards for 100 days, cadmium for 5 days, inorganic mercury for 100 days and methyl mercury for 60 days.

I have gone into some detail in my efforts to explain the benefits of this purification compound, because I feel that it is invaluable as a cleansing agent. I believe that the manufacturers of BRIMAC 216 have achieved a marvellous objective and I wish to express my gratitude for the information they have so freely supplied to me. It is with thanks to them that I can advise some of my patients accordingly.

Pure water has become a rare commodity in our modern world. Every day I look with gratitude at the spring water feeding the small lake near my house and marvel at the clarity and purity of the water that comes down from the hills. This water has not been tampered with and contains a wealth of minerals and trace elements — and it still tastes as water should. However, with trepidation I wonder how long this water will remain as pure as it is at present, taking into consideration the atmospheric influences at work. I do not doubt that in time to come the quality of the water will be affected, and I do not know how to stop the contamination of the spring. We must be aware of what can be carried along in the water and what we can do to avoid contamination. This is one of the reasons I was so pleased to learn about the charcoal filter described above.

In relation to the subject of cleansers, I must point out that the most marvellous cleansers of impurities in our body are the kidneys. These days our kidneys must be badly overworked in their capacity as a filtering system. Just think of the filters in an air-conditioning system or of the exhaust fumes from industrial plants and factories which must be channelled off. Our kidneys are constantly called upon to rid our body of toxic waste, and with the aid of the liver they perform a marvellous function. If the kidneys could not cope with the task that has been demanded of them, uraemia would set in within a short time and the functions of other important organs in the body would be severely impaired as a result. It has been calculated that under normal circumstances the kidneys are required to filter approximately 60 litres of urine a day. After the filtering process that takes place in the kidneys, the urine is separated and transported to the bladder, from where it will be discharged by way of the urethra.

Most people have sufficient understanding of the body to realise how vital the functions of the kidneys are and therefore we should do our best not to be too demanding of them. A high intake of salt and toxic materials will severely increase their workload and there is no doubt that permanent impairment of the kidneys will be detrimental to our general health. In this context we would do well to consider the damage that could be caused by some of the high metal contents found in some sources of water.

Metallic poisons are notoriously threatening to our health. Some particular people, whose work makes them more vulnerable, are advised to take care to prevent the situation getting out of hand. I have seen many badly arthritic patients for whom lead poisoning was certainly a contributory cause of their condition, e.g. taxi drivers, long-distance lorry drivers, people who work in the printing industry who have been exposed to printing ink fumes, or painters. If your daily occupation poses risks to your kidneys, do take care. To nourish our kidneys it is helpful to drink certain herbal teas, for example *Solidago* (goldenrod), on a regular basis. However, the most marvellous remedy in this case is *Harpagophytum*, an extract from a root by the same name, also known as devil's claw. For metabolic dysfunctions, rheumatism, arthritis, liver, gallbladder, kidney and bladder problems, this is one of the best remedies I can recommend. Moreover, it is also effective in cases of allergic reactions. If the urine is cloudy or smells stronger than normal, pay attention to this and drink larger quantities of water to flush through and so cleanse the kidneys. But do make sure that the water you use is pure.

A little while ago I met a remarkable 98-year-old lady. Her mental faculties were totally unimpaired and physically, too, she was in very good shape. Imagine my surprise when I discovered that she did not require glasses even for reading. This she accredited to the fact that her mother had insisted that every day she use an eye bath of lukewarm water with one or two drops of *Euphrasia* (eyebright) added. She had adhered to this habit all her life and faithfully believed that this was the reason for her perfect eyesight. She also told me that whenever she feels the onset of a cold which might result in some congestion, she immediately uses an old-fashioned nasal spray, which she fills with salt water. She is indeed a remarkable lady.

The great physician Boerhaeve (1688-1738) maintained that we should always endeavour to 'keep the head cool, the feet warm and the bowel as empty as possible'. When Dr Vogel and I opened the first naturopathic clinic in the Netherlands in 1959 we were advised by a very knowledgeable person, Dr ten Haaf, to install an apparatus for bowel cleansing. Apparently, way back in 1935, he had a chair bowel bath in his clinic in Germany and thousands of patients underwent this cleansing treatment. We followed his advice and installed and used this rather complicated apparatus. Sometimes, as much as 5 litres of water would be used per application per patient. The feedback from our patients was as enthusiastic as Dr ten Haaf led us to expect. There were actually instances when we had to inform a patient that it was not advisable to undergo this treatment on a daily basis, as their bowels had to be encouraged to perform the task for themselves.

Young babies who are not fed any solids, but are still breastfed or obtain their nourishment from bottled milk, produce a soiled nappy after most feeds. This is a sign of good bowel movement. The baby has taken those nutrients from the food it requires and the rest is quickly discharged from the body. In adulthood this pattern changes to one motion a day and even that is by no means the case for every adult.

I remember listening to a lecture in Canada by the well-known practitioner Mike Carson, in which he told his audience about the efficacy of a coffee enema. He made no bones about it, but told the gathering that to his way of thinking if coffee was enjoyed in the acceptable manner it was being entered at the wrong end, because the benefits would be much greater if it were to be administered as an enema. Indeed, it is often surprising to hear people's reactions once they have tried an enema treatment. Most of them maintain that the good feeling they experience afterwards more than outweighs any temporary inconvenience.

Also for irrigation of the bowels it is possible to use water that has been heated to the approximate temperature of 40 °C (104 °F) with the juice of half a lemon added. However, to my mind the most successful enema is obtained using tea that has been infused from the bark of the oak tree. Use 2 litres of water with two tablespoons of oak bark extract; irrigation with this will produce some excellent results. To cleanse the body of parasites such as ringworm or threadworm, the onion treatment is invaluable. Boil 1 kilogram of chopped onions in 2 litres of water. Allow this to cool down and then strain before using the resulting extract as an enema. This is a wonderful way to rid the body of foreign invaders. In the case of children make sure that the child is given lots of carrots to eat the day prior to the treatment, and if possible some coconut. Even chronic infestations of worms can be eliminated with this treatment.

Every now and then we are given to understand that medical innovations and developments have come to the end of the road. Nothing could be further from the truth. We must continue our search for the most effective forms of treatment, and in this context water plays a very important role. Some of the old treatment methods are still as effective as ever, yet this does not mean that we cannot improve on them. My main concern is that we should try to follow the rules of nature as closely as we can; by doing so we will not go far wrong.

6

Water as Medicine

FATHER SEBASTIAN KNEIPP (1821-97), a Dominican priest, was in his time considered a most remarkable person, whose life was more dedicated to saving lives than to the salvation of souls. He became more and more engrossed in the application of water treatments and pioneered this field zealously. He advised his parishioners to walk barefoot in the fields while the dew was still on the grass and to paddle in the little stream. His ideas on water therapy turned out to be so effective in practice that he became very widely known. Money streamed in from grateful patients and with this revenue he built three large clinics, the most famous of which, Kneipp Spa, housed more than 7,000 beds.

Father Kneipp used water as a medicine, and quite a few of his treatments are still used today with equally satisfying results. Occasionally I have heard criticism of his methods, but then again the criticism was not aimed at their effectiveness, but on the fact that some of the means were less than pleasant. However, Father Kneipp developed many different forms of treatment — either active or passive, some combined with diet and others incorporating the use of herbs — and the popularity of his methods must be considered sufficient evidence of his success. Father Kneipp's understanding was well ahead of his time, as through his treatment formulae he aimed to give the body a certain measure of immunity against unforeseen circumstances, i.e. to boost the body's immune system.

Long before Father Kneipp, however, the farmer Vincenz Priestnitz, who was born in 1799 in Silesia, was also working with water cures, and he too was widely known. Like Kneipp, Priestnitz was never a great advocate of showers. Both of them much preferred to use sitz baths or a total bath, especially if the treatment was supposed to take place towards the end of the day. Occasionally they would recommend a good body wash to be finished off by pouring water over the body with the aid of a container. In those days water cures or treatments were mainly applied for complaints such as colds, bronchitis, catarrh, colic and cramp, and the recommendation then would be to relax in a hot bath of a temperature around 40 °C (104 °F) for 10-15 minutes. Where an older patient was concerned, especially when a heart problem was also suspected, both Kneipp and Priestnitz would recommend a lukewarm bath instead. Where a very cold sitz bath or a full bath treatment was indicated, this was limited to only five seconds and after such a bath the use of a towel was discouraged; instead, the patient would be advised to dress before the skin was fully dry. In cases of colic or circulatory problems, Father Kneipp would advise taking a small sitz bath at a temperature of approximately 40 °C (104 °F) for no longer than fifteen minutes.

Father Kneipp advocated several different ways of taking foot baths. The alternate hot and cold foot bath — to be repeated twice — was a special favourite of his. Cold foot baths were not to last longer than one minute and here water could be trickled down the back of the legs.

It was always recommended that cool water be used for an eye bath. Sometimes it was suggested that cool compresses be placed on the eyes for about thirty seconds. Please note that the water used should never be ice-cold.

If you suffer from cold hands or numb fingers, you would be well advised to immerse the limbs in hot water (approximately 40 °C/104 °F) for anything up to ten minutes and then quickly run cold water over them for about ten seconds. This is to be repeated twice.

Of course drinking water is also therapeutically important. Never forget that the organs are cleansed by drinking water. It also serves to dilute other liquids present in the body, cleanse the cells, lower the body temperature and stimulate the circulation. Particularly in cases of diabetes it is important to drink sufficient quantities and I have already noted the need for people with kidney problems to do this. Diabetics are advised to drink at least 6-8 glasses of pure water every day. In order to stimulate the liver or to solve constipation problems a larger-than-average intake of water is important too. People who suffer from constipation are specifically advised to drink at least two glasses of cold water before breakfast and this advice is also applicable to rheumatic people. For common colds one should also drink more than average to replenish the body fluids; variety may be introduced by drinking herbal teas during the day. If you are troubled with gallstones, drink as many as twelve glasses of water — preferably bottled water. People who are trying to counteract their addiction to alcohol or other drugs should also remember that plenty of body fluids are required to cleanse the system of their poisonous effects.

I am the proud owner of a very old book on Father Kneipp's cures, *Wie Kneipp Kur — Warum und Wann? (Who Should Have a Kneipp Cure — Where and When?)*, and it is encouraging to see that although he largely advocated the use of water as a remedy, he also recommended certain herbal concoctions and, among other herbs, chamomile is listed regularly. The therapeutic value of water added to the remedial effects of certain herbs definitely make a powerful combination. He treated adults and children alike with these remedies, and the one I describe below was always reputed to have been very successful in reducing fevers in children. This remedy will of course work equally well for adults, but it is worth remembering that children can very quickly develop an extreme change in their body temperature, whereas this will occur more gradually in adults.

Prepare an infusion using equal parts of salt, cider vinegar and, if available, some thyme, chamomile, fennel and lime blossom. Seat the child on a large towel and then divide the mixture between several compresses to be placed on the chest and back of the child. Cover everything with some warm towels. The temperature will soon come down and the treatment may be repeated several times during the day or night, as required.

In similar circumstances Kneipp's unique treatment was to dissolve two cups of table salt in about 2 litres of cold water. Wash the child with this water before dressing him in a pre-warmed cotton garment and putting him to bed.

For stomach problems I have already mentioned the usefulness of chamomile compresses, but you may like to know that Centaurium will serve equally well for this purpose.

One of Kneipp's favourite treatments was to collect some juniper berries and rosehips and, if available, some oat-straw and/or horsetail. The herbs were infused in some boiling water and, after straining, this infusion would be stirred into the hot bath water. This therapy was highly recommended when the patient had urinary problems. It is a useful one to know as it is always difficult to find good diuretics that can be taken without having to suffer from unpleasant side-effects. This is not only the case in natural medicine, but is even more true of orthodox medicine. Do not forget that water in itself is an excellent diuretic, and one that can be used even if one feels obliged to also follow a course of chemical diuretics.

Hot compresses, saunas and Turkish baths are all important in treating such problems. Also, as an alternative to water, Dr Vogel's herbal kidney tea may be used, which is an excellent natural diuretic. My own grandmother worked out a combination of sixteen different herbs, which is available today as a herbal health tea and is completely safe to use in the treatment of a wide range of different health problems. This tea is now marketed worldwide and has been found effective in relieving the suffering of many people.

The concept that water may be utilised as a medicine has probably been around as long as mankind. A visit to a spa was an essential part of the social calendar during the last century, and even the royal family would take time off for this. Today, millions of people from all over the world make their pilgrimage to Lourdes to drink the water. Here again nature has provided us with water that is endowed with many natural gifts. The properties of the mineral germanium has recently been given much publicity in the scientific world and this mineral is found in abundance in the water at Lourdes. Germanium has been found to be of tremendous value in alleviating degenerative diseases, and for those people who find relief at Lourdes, water can indeed be regarded as miraculous!

Not only in Lourdes but also in Japan there are centres where the waters are rich in germanium and are claimed to have medicinal properties. According to folklore, many other countries have their own sources of 'healing' water as, indeed, is true of Britain. These waterfalls or wells are unusually rich in minerals and trace elements, which accounts for the fact that the water is endowed with medicinal characteristics. I have become particularly interested in a certain source of water in Wales, which has been used for medicinal purposes for centuries. Although this source has always existed, it has been receiving greater publicity in recent years and is now becoming more widely known. It is considered beneficial to both drink and bathe in this water

— and if there was ever any doubt that water could possess 'remedial properties', then this water would certainly dispel them. I myself have seen people with serious anaemic problems whose condition was clearly reversed after drinking water from this source in Wales, namely the Trefriw Wells.

Fortunately, the water from this source is now being bottled and has become much more widely available. It is marketed under the name of 'Trefriw Wells Roman Spa Water', and is recognised by many as being of great benefit to people who suffer from a wide variety of health conditions, such as anaemia, rheumatism, lumbago, nervous tension, mental fatigue, loss of energy, depression, skin complaints and muscular aches. This water is carefully bottled with nothing being added or taken away from it, so that it remains completely natural. Many people have testified that an eight-week course has brought about a change for the better in their health.

The reason I became interested in this particular spa was that in my experience it is one of the richest sources of minerals and trace elements that exists. The water obtained from Trefriw Wells can also be described as 'chalybeate' spa water, the word 'chalybeate' meaning 'iron in solution', and it is the only spa water of its type that is known to exist in the protosulphate form, enabling it to be bottled for use at home. The water is supplied in small actinic bottles to ensure that it remains fresh during use and hence retains its high potency. It is quite wonderful to think that this spa water is now widely available to the public, and can be obtained in many of the better health food stores and chemists.

Today's hectic lifestyle, coupled with an excess of convenience foods in many cases, encourages mineral deficiencies. This water, rich in iron, combined with other essential minerals in a most easily digested, active — and therefore powerful — form, makes an ideal natural dietary supplement to replace some of these deficiencies and tone up the whole system. Iron is, without question, one of the most crucial elements for ensuring optimum health, since it directly affects the oxygen-carrying capacity of the blood by increasing the quantity of red corpuscles that carry oxygen to the body tissues and vital organs. The following analysis of this water is given as a brief guide to some of the uses our body can make of the minerals contained in Trefriw Wells Spa Water, when they are present in our body in the correct amounts:

Minerals

Iron   In the haemoglobin, acts as an oxygen carrier in the red blood cells. In the myoglobin, acts as an oxygen reservoir in the muscles.

Sulphur   A mild laxative.

Silica   An essential component of cartilage, important for strength and elasticity of gristle. Helps to keep the arterial walls elastic. Controls the uptake of calcium. Also an important factor in the regulation of blood pressure.

Calcium   Builds and maintains healthy bones and teeth. Helps to control the excitability of the nerves and muscles. Helps the blood to control its cholesterol levels. Acts as a detoxifying agent in relation to lead, mercury and cadmium.

Potassium An essential activator in a number of enzymes, particularly those concerned with energy production.

Magnesium A co-factor in many body processes, including energy and cell replication. Responsible for the formation of strong, decay-resistant tooth enamel.

Sodium   Important for maintaining a normal balance of water between body cells and the surrounding fluids. (Potassium also contributes to this.)

Trace Elements

Manganese   Important for the development and maintenance of a healthy nervous system and the maintenance of healthy bones. A co-factor for energy production and the health of joints.

Zinc   Important for a healthy liver function, growth and insulin production.

Chromium   Acts as a glucose tolerance factor (GTF) in combination with other substances, i.e. controls the level of blood glucose by promoting its uptake by the muscles and organs and stimulating the burning of glucose for energy. Reduces fat levels in the blood.

Copper   Important for blood formation, in that it aids iron absorption and incorporation into haemoglobin. A co-factor for many enzymes, e.g. those needed for skin healing and those that protect the body from toxic agents.

It was between the years AD 90 and 250 when the soldiers of the Roman Empire first realised the value of the spa waters and tunnelled into the Allt Coch mountain in Wales to obtain the liquid as it rose through fissures in the rock. Since that time the chalybeate spa water from Trefriw Wells has been used as a natural aid to healthy living by countless people from all over the world, and it still benefits people today.

Before I proceed to another topic, I will relate a poem that I came across, written in 1911 by a grateful patient, in praise of the Trefriw waters as a specific cure for insomnia:

> *To Trefriw Wells, a lady came—*
> *(Her nerves all shattered) — old and lame.*
> *Her joy of life and spirits spent,*
> *Her days were just one long lament*
> *Against the wretched motor-man,*
> *Who knocked her down with a span.*

This shock to nerves caused sleeplessness;
The broken arm gave hopelessness;
With bruises, cuts and all contusions
She listened to her friends' effusions,
To join them in the loveliest spot
That loving nature e'er begot.

To drink the Water from the Wells,
(Which pain and anguish, quickly quells),
She came. She drank. The baths she tried.
And sleep returned, so long denied:
Had she the ready writer's flow,
This wondrous cure, all men should know.

Two or three years ago I attended a conference on cancer research held in Los Angeles. I was invited by one of my colleagues to accompany her to a lecture on a certain water that was claimed to have remedial properties and was currently receiving considerable acclaim in the United States. I cannot say that the lecture was especially stimulating and, unfortunately, I was not giving it my full attention. However, I had heard enough to make me look through the handouts after the lecture, and when I realised the mineral and trace element content of the water, I felt compelled to look into it further. Again, it appeared that one of the most outstanding features of the water was its high germanium content. Germanium is also found in a few plants, e.g. aloe, comfrey and garlic, but this water came from the Black Hills of South Dakota, and before surfacing passed through the natural filtering process of a coalmine. The water has been marketed in the United States under the name of 'Dr Willard's' and is also known as 'Catalyst Altered Water' — and many, many people have been willing to vouch for its curative properties.

In 1980 a Select Committee on Ageing drawn from the US House of Representatives met in order to give their approval to Catalyst Altered Water and I will quote here the self-explanatory introduction given by the Chairperson of the Select Committee, followed by a resumé of the statement made by Professor John Willard, PhD.

We are here to discuss a substance called Catalyst Altered Water. It is best known by several other names, such as LA water or Lignite Activated Water, but for today's session, we'll refer to the broader term of Catalyst Altered Water.

The water was brought to my attention a few months ago following a hearing by the House Ageing Committee on DMSO — a controversial substance which has been claimed effective against arthritis and a number of other ailments. Upon investigation of the issues, I found that hundreds of South Dakotans, including many elderly persons, have been using Catalyst Altered Water on a regular basis.

We have heard that people have been using the water for everything from warts to cancer, and that many of the elderly have used it on a continual basis for chronic health problems. Since 81 per cent of all persons over 65 suffer from one or more chronic conditions, these people are especially likely to seek out promised cures like Catalyst Altered Water. Consequently, it is imperative that we know more about this substance.

I have no idea whether Catalyst Altered Water is the 'Miracle Cure' that many have claimed it to be, but I do think it is our responsibility to bring it forward for closer scrutiny. If the water does indeed have the potential for treating ailments, we need to encourage further study and expedite its approval for human use. If the substance is effective, it is important that those individuals who have been buying and using it are given the best information possible.

I am not in a position to judge the medical or therapeutic merits of Catalyst Altered Water, and we don't intend to resolve that question today. This is an exploratory hearing during which we want to ask a few basic questions:

—What is Catalyst Altered Water and how is it developed?
—How many people are using the water, and what are they using it for?
—How is it marketed?
—Is there any scientifically valid evidence that shows Catalyst Altered Water to be effective in preventing or treating ailments?
—Is Catalyst Altered Water potentially harmful?

In addition to these questions, we intend to examine the issue of regulation and approval of new drugs for human use. For regulatory purposes, Catalyst Altered Water is considered a drug, and as such, it would require approval by the Food and Drug Administration before being marketed for human use.

Some have claimed that the Food and Drug Administration regulations hinder the development of new drugs by forcing the inventor to invest millions of dollars and years of time obtaining approval from the FDA. Just a month ago, the General Accounting Office released a report entitled 'FDA approval — A lengthy process that delays the availability of important new drugs'. It is important to review the impact of that process on independent researchers like Dr Willard who do not have the benefit of large, well-funded laboratories.

Have FDA requirements been effective in uncovering the safety and usefulness of unknown substances? Have they interfered with the development and marketing of potentially beneficial drugs? How have they influenced the development of Catalyst Altered Water in particular? Those questions will be addressed today with the help of Food and Drug Administration officials from Washington.

We have an excellent line-up of witnesses today, and I look forward to hearing their testimony. . . . The first witness is Dr John Willard, the producer of Catalyst Altered Water. I'd like to hear his comments.

Statement of John Willard, PhD, Professor Emeritus, South Dakota School of Mines and Technology, Department of Chemistry, Rapid City, South Dakota:

Catalyst Altered Water is nothing more or less than ordinary water that has been modified by a catalyst that I happened to develop. We have a form that is much more reactive than water. This Catalyst Altered Water is something I stumbled on trying to prove to my son that I could do something that he said I couldn't. And in trying to prove to him that I could do it, I did it, which is the history of things scientific. This Catalyst Altered Water gives a more reactive form of water. When you look at this planet earth, this is a water world. Three-quarters of its surface is probably covered with water. All living things, at least on the surface of the earth, are water-oriented. Man himself spends time in his mother's womb as a sea animal up until the time the water breaks. Then he becomes an oxygen-breathing animal. So this is true: 68 per cent of our bodies right now is water. The young of the species may go up to 90 or 95 per cent. It is essential for the growth of all plants and animals, and we can see from the present drought when crops are not doing well and the animals are dying, that water is essential on this planet earth. But still, the regulatory agencies across the country, both state and national, will not admit that water is a nutrient. When you figure that 68 per cent of every pound produced is water, I don't see how they . . . well, water is too complex. So that is the history and background of the water. . . .

The Catalyst Altered Water is obtained by changing the chemical structure of water. We start with a sodium silicate, which some of the older people remember as water glass. We used to preserve eggs in it, a few years before we had refrigeration. We use calcium chloride, which is quite commonly used to settle dust on the roads. I use magnesium sulphate, which is Epsom salts. All these in small amounts, and then I use a castor oil. Those are the basic ingredients, but they are combined with an art, so that it makes a caloric particle, which has an intense electrical field surrounding it, so that it will polarise water, and place it in an arrangement of water molecules to each other in space that makes it much more reactive. Now it might be informative if we see how the arrangement of component particles such as atoms, ions and molecules determine the properties of matter. We have the colloidal, with a deep carbon atom bonded to four other carbon atoms three dimensionally. Ordinarily, water has the same structure: one water molecule bonded to four, and each one of those to four, and so on and on. And that's why water is the shape that we have it. If this were not so, water should be a gas at 60° below zero. Now I could go back to the carbon system with the graphite. If we convert, and we can, a diamond, and put it under stress, so that each carbon, instead of bonding to four others, would bond to only three, then we have graphite, which is soft enough that we can use it in lead pencils. We use it as a lubricant. Now my catalyst, to the best of our knowledge, does the same thing with water. We have a graphite form of liquid water, and the properties are as much different from ordinary water as graphite is from the diamond. . . .

The basic Catalyst Altered Water is used in a diluted form. Because I had been interested in lignite coal when I came from the mines in 1946, after I got my family settled, I started looking around to see what was in the state that was paying my salary, so that I could benefit the state. I have a sense of feeling that all of us ought to do what we can to better mankind. And my philosophy is that there is three-quarters of a million tons of lignite coal within 500 miles of Rapid City. . . . And here we have these tons of coal, which are the fossil remains of plants and trees that grew 50 million years ago . . . and I tried to find out how we could use this material for something other than a fuel. I find in the literature that for 300 years scientists have been trying to unlock this wealth. Once I got the basic idea of Catalyst Altered Water, with my research it suddenly became possible that I could take lignite coal and, reacting it with the water (incidentally this water is so harmless that we can drink and bathe in it, but still it will tear the coal apart), releasing the wealth, then destroying the phenols and the toxic materials, the carcinogens, which are in ordinary coal. Then it becomes water soluble. . . . We make four or five different products, but they are basically the same. It's just a matter of the different concentrations, and the uses we put them to. . . .

First we tested if there's any toxic material, and if it could be harmful in any way. I have about four different analyses by reputable laboratories — and they were testing the concentrated form, which is never used, because we use the diluted form. Now as far as the clinical testing which scientists do, we have not done it for one reason — I didn't have the money to do such research. And as a retired professor of chemistry, I realised that our testing was done under carefully controlled conditions, and not really related to the real world, where conditions are not ideal. So I've done most of my testing with ranchers and farmers and nurses and doctors and people like that, under real conditions. I will admit that this is not accepted by scientists in the community because you don't have quality controls. But every human, every animal, is different, so how can you run a control when you can't find two identical species? . . .

Catalyst Altered Water was tested by the WARF Institute — an Alumni Research Foundation, approved by the FDA. There it was tested for everything — for toxic materials, whether there were carcinogens in there to cause cancer. They tested it to see if there was mutation, any basic change, in cell structure, and they gave us a clean bill of health. . . .

The hearing then continued with a number of case histories and the evidence of witnesses who had used Catalyst Altered Water and had benefited from it. I will not go into any further detail here, but let me tell you that the testimonies recorded make very impressive reading.

Let us move on now to Salzburg in Austria, where the Gasteiner Heilstollen can be found. This is a fascinating spa, where modern comforts are combined with local knowledge of the medicinal properties of the water in that area. A tastefully decorated clinic has been established in these beautiful surroundings in the healthy mountain air. A unique tunnelling system in the mountain allows patients to participate in thermal baths, exercises, underwater exercises, etc. — and all this takes place within carefully controlled levels of humidity and temperature. Due to the warmth and humidity of the atmosphere the patients are better able to benefit from the water, which has a favourable influence on the metabolic functioning of the cells.

Our outlook on life is strongly influenced by the environment in which we live, although seldom would we agree with that statement. Most of us would think twice about paddling, let alone bathing, in muddy water. Yet that is exactly what the South American Indians, among others, do. Similarly, in the lakes of Scandinavia the water can be what we would politely call a 'less attractive' colour, yet people will still bathe in it. In the spring this water will, in fact, be freshly melted snow, which will have gushed down in little streams from the mountains before collecting in the lakes. Some of the silt deposits from the mountains will have rushed along with the stream and it is most probable that it is these deposits that give the water its medicinal properties. The quality and characteristics of water will vary according to its source, as they will each have been subjected to different electric fields.

Bathing in sea water can also be extremely beneficial and the stories we hear about medicinal properties obtained from the water of the Dead Sea are quite astounding. As I have mentioned earlier, in cases of psoriasis — this skin disease that is so difficult to cure — Dead Sea water has brought tremendous relief, and for this reason a large clinic has been established on the shores of the Dead Sea, where dermatologists take care of people from all over the world who are desperate to find a cure for their psoriasis.

I would like to mention here another extremely capable person in the field of hydrotherapy, Louis Kuehne. He has written many books on hydrotherapy and even though these have been translated into many languages, I still feel it is a great pity that his methods have not received more acclaim. He has devised various water treatments which have proved to be very successful. One of these involves the patient sitting in a three-quarters full cold sitz bath. The patient then rubs and brushes the genitals using a towel in a circular motion. When practising this treatment it is important to keep the upper half of the body as warm as possible. Once the patient has conditioned himself to continuing this treatment for a full five minutes at a time, the benefits will become obvious by a greatly improved feeling of general well-being.

In the Far East serious problems such as gangrene are treated with similar therapies. Warm-water compresses to which certain herbs are added are gently but persistently rubbed onto the affected area. This treatment activates the leucocytes and lymphocytes and also overcomes blood-clotting and stimulates the discharge of poisonous substances. All in all, this type of treatment is excellent for any metabolic disorder.

Another effective treatment for metabolic disorders is as follows. First, spread a rubber or plastic sheet over the bed and cover this with a sheet that has been soaked in cold water. The patient then drinks a glass of hot tea with lemon juice, sweetened with a little soft brown sugar. If preferred, some herbal health tea may be taken.

The second part of this treatment requires the patient to pass water.

In the third phase, the patient has a shower or a sponge bath, after which he should lie down on the cold, wet sheet, cover himself with some blankets and place a cold cloth over his forehead. It is helpful if the patient has some company at this stage, because he is supposed to remain in this position for an hour. If he were to have a temperature, this is bound to disappear and he will relax totally.

For the fourth and final phase of the treatment the patient has a lukewarm shower, without towelling dry afterwards. He should then relax and take things easy.

A large quantity of body liquid will have been eliminated during this procedure and sometimes the perspiration resulting from this treatment may well be unpleasant to the nostrils, but this should be viewed as an indication that the patient will have got rid of much toxic material from the body. This is an old-fashioned method which will help anybody who is not feeling well. You can also add some chamomile to the water in which the sheet is soaked. It is also possible to adapt this method for application to a specific limb or other part of the body, in which case the treatment will be restricted to a local therapy.

For relief from toothache or a migraine, fold a compress to approximately the size of a gent's handkerchief, wet this in cold water and place it on the relevant area, leaving it in place for 20-30 minutes. The same can be done for chest problems, in which case it will be important to place a hot towel over the compress. The same size of compress can be used for liver or gallbladder problems, but then it should be covered by a warm woollen cloth. In such cases, however, the treatment will be more beneficial if the compress is hot — not so hot as to scald the body of course. For localised treatment of the stomach area, the size of the compress may be slightly increased.

An effective way of using water as a medicine is the old-fashioned drink cure. To successfully eliminate toxins from the body the patient should fast for two days and drink at least 2-3 litres of water per day. For this cure it would be preferable to use distilled water. Especially if the patient is due to follow a cure over the next two or three weeks, this is an ideal way to cleanse the body in advance.

The Russians, Finns and North Americans tend to be great believers in sweat baths. In preparation, it is advisable to drink at least half a litre of herbal tea; either chamomile or elderflower is recommended for this purpose. The bath should be filled with water at a good hot temperature and the bathroom should also be kept warm. In the olden days a steam bath would be taken in a wooden cupboard or box and it would be arranged in such a way that the head would stick out of the cupboard. Nowadays, a much easier and more enjoyable way to obtain the benefits of a sweat bath is to have a Turkish bath, which is ideal for this purpose and affords a marvellous opportunity for relaxation afterwards.

The eyes are very responsive to sensible water treatment and an eye bath to which has been added a few drops of Dr Vogel's Euphrasiasan will take away any tiredness. This will also give great relief in cases of conjunctivitis.

I will describe one of my grandmother's favourite treatments for cases of mouth or throat infections. First, use water that has been heated to the temperature of 37 °C (98.6 °F) and then have some more water ready at a temperature of 23 °C (73.4 °F). Use the warmer water first as a gargle, to be followed by the cooler water. Add one or two teaspoons of hydrogen peroxide 3 per cent to the second glass; if preferred, the hydrogen peroxide may be replaced by some salt, lemon or *Salvia*. In most cases you will find that mouth ulcers or other oral infections will disappear quickly using this treatment.

Nasal problems may be treated with a nose brush, which is available from chemists, but it is even better to rinse the nose with salt water. Sniff this water high up into the nose and nasal congestion will soon disappear.

Having expounded the benefits of water as a medicine, let us not forget the comfort to be obtained from the use of ice. The most gratifying treatment with ice must be when I show an asthmatic patient how to place an ice-cube on the dorsal spine, between the fourth and fifth vertebrae, in order to obtain fast and effective relief during moments of anxiety.

Among my patients I count many sports personalities and many a time I have used ice packs to arrest or reduce initial bruising or swellings. I have even resorted to the use of ice-cubes for broken bones. The cold treatment will arrest internal bleeding as well as reduce the pain. Occasionally, I have even given a patient an ice massage. Unlike some practitioners, I have never been very much in favour of heat treatment in cases of inflammation or acute trauma. In my experience much more benefit is to be gained from the use of ice-cubes or ice-cold water treatments in those circumstances. Take an ordinary rubber hot-water bottle, fill this with ice-cubes, crushed slightly if necessary, and return it to the freezer compartment. This will provide you with an effective home treatment for painful joints, headaches, swellings, and can even be used as a home anaesthetic.

The so-called ICE therapy, meaning *Ice Compression* and *Elevation*, is tremendous for sports injuries. As soon as possible after the injury has occurred ice-cubes are placed on the affected part and kept in place by a bandage. An elastic bandage is then placed over the top for light compression. This will greatly reduce the pain and bring speedy relief. However, do not apply this treatment more than three times a day. With a bit of ingenuity, a larger or more specific area can be treated with the ICE therapy, by devising compresses, hats or suits for different purposes. While the cold compresses are being refreshed, briefly alternate the treatment with some lukewarm compresses.

Not long ago, I was consulted by a patient who was greatly troubled by kidney problems. She was suffering a great deal of discomfort and I instructed her to drink as much water as she could manage, and to take some *Solidago* (goldenrod) three times daily. Instead of tea or coffee she was to drink herbal tea and I specifically recommended the rosehip variety or beechleaf tea. The result was totally satisfying. This lady had been informed that surgery to remove her kidney stones was unavoidable. However, she followed my advice and spontaneously discharged the stones. Water treatment once again had proved victorious.

It happens every now and then that a patient runs a temperature for no apparent reason. In the first instance, then, the aim must be to reduce the temperature; for this purpose use the method I described on page 37. Parmenides — the father of metaphysics — is quoted as having said: 'Give me the power to raise the temperature and I will heal every illness.' Indeed, it is often the case that when the fever reaches its crisis, some of these unidentified diseases will disappear once the body gets rid of the toxins or alien material it contained.

I would like to think that in this chapter I have given you sufficient reasons to appreciate the power of water as a medicine.

7

Spa Water

IT WAS WITH FULL sympathy that I regarded the man opposite me who had a nervous look about him. Wringing his hands, he tensely watched the equipment he was in charge of. He had been instructed to drill in an area in the north of the Dutch province of Limburg where, according to geological reports, there ought to be a rich source of mineral water. At a depth of 800 metres, nothing yet . . . 830 metres . . . 850 metres . . . still nothing. Then, suddenly, at a depth of 856 metres a spout of water sprang up around the drill with tremendous force. In accordance with the geological reports, we had hit a rich supply of mineral water, and I say rich because subsequent investigation of this water confirmed that it contained a wealth of minerals. Since then, the water has proved to be of value in the treatment of rheumatism, arthritis and psoriasis, and many people are prepared to attest to the benefits of the water at the thermal baths in Arcen, North Limburg, in the Netherlands.

Every time I visit there, which recently has been quite often, I look at the many visitors and patients, more than a few of them crippled for various reasons. Without exception they are pleased to tell me about the benefits of the water at the thermal baths and, in particular, claim that the combination of the heat and the quality of the water has improved their condition.

We can only be grateful that this source of water was eventually discovered, but why did we have to drill so deep? The sources of water at some of the spas that were so popular in the last century were generally found on the surface, and certainly nowhere were they as deep as we had to drill in Arcen. Unfortunately, many of these once well-attended resorts have since been closed owing to lack of interest. Yet their waters were of equal remedial value. Britain had its share of well-known spas and many people were in the habit of visiting them once a year or more often. They would arrange to meet their friends or relatives and 'take the waters' together in well-known places such as Bath, Harrogate, Tunbridge Wells or Brighton in England, the Trefriw Wells in Wales, and Crieff, Peebles and Strathpeffer in Scotland — to name but a few. In many of these spa towns the social life flourished in accordance with the amount of visitors they received and theatres opened rapidly to ensure that the valued customers would be entertained during their stay. Dressmakers were kept busy because the ladies had to show off their finery at the many dinners given in honour of the various celebrities. Parents would take their eligible offspring along in the hope that some valuable introductions could be made for the future. Public transport in and to these towns was second to none, even though the upper classes would usually bring their own transport with them. High-class hotels and elegant town houses were built to accommodate the influx of visitors, and libraries and other facilities were opened. In short, the public and social life in these towns thrived.

How unfortunate it is that the habit of 'taking the waters' has been allowed to die out, when it provided so many benefits. Even as far back as 1320 it was reported that the local iron-master was cured in the town spa near Liège in Belgium after drinking the iron-rich chalybeate water. (Remember, 'chalybeate' water means water saturated with iron salts.) Well before that time, the Romans drank the water and they knew the effects of drinking such water and bathing in it. In the year 1735 patients flocked from far and wide to visit the various spas which had become well known because of their medicinal values, but little did they know that it was because of the various chemical salts in those waters that their joints ached less. By 1745 English ladies had become almost different creatures; they were more relaxed and took as many of these water treatments as possible.

The Crieff Hydro in Scotland was founded in 1868 and today is still (or rather, again) a much sought-after place to 'take the waters'. The recent revival in interest in water treatments has led to it being developed further. It is the same in Germany, Switzerland and Austria, where once-popular spas have lately been reopened to enable people to bathe in as well as drink these curative waters. The same pattern has also been repeated at Trefriw Wells in Wales which, as I described earlier, have been reopened to begin a new chapter in their already great history.

Dr Doby of Chester, who in his day was a highly regarded physician, wrote to the Rt. Hon. W. E. Gladstone:

> I have no hesitation in saying that the Trefriw waters are among the finest chalybeate waters in this or any other country. Amongst my patients I have witnessed very remarkable curative effects since they took the Trefriw waters. I have visited and examined most of the celebrated establishments in Germany, so I think that I may speak with some confidence on this point.

Another physician concluded:

> It is therefore the best of sulphate chalybeate water to be found in Great Britain.

It is with good reason that the Trefriw Wells Roman Spa Water is considered an excellent dietary supplement for toning up the whole system and, in a general sense, assisting in the treatment of a wide range of conditions such as anaemia, rheumatism, nervous tension, depression, mental fatigue, various skin complaints and several other chronic conditions. Thanks to the minerals found in this water we can also obtain a measure of immunity against the usual winter ailments. The Roman soldiers who discovered the source of this curative water recognised it for what it was when they were prospecting for minerals in the Welsh mountains. These soldiers were driven extremely hard by their superiors in their search for supremacy and their quest to conquer unknown territories. Centuries later, the cave was re-excavated as interest in water treatments was revived. The Trefriw Wells are situated in the most captivating countryside; indeed, most spas are to be found amid beautiful surroundings. Interest in the water at Trefriw Wells increased considerably during the latter part of the nineteenth century and a grand bathing complex was established.

Today, the beneficial characteristics of this water can be captured in bottled form thanks to modern science and, therefore, many more people can avail themselves of this water that is so rich in curative properties. Results may be attained within a fairly short period and for many people a single eight-week graduated course is sufficient. Others may require two or even three courses. Some people also find it beneficial to extend the period during which they use the more concentrated solution until they achieve the required results. Although it is not necessary to use the spa water continuously, it may be desirable to follow up the intensive treatment with a daily supplement. Alternatively, it may be suggested that an eight-week course be taken two or three times a year, at the change of seasons for example. Always remember that the water can be taken alongside prescribed medication without any danger of side-effects, and this in itself is a great advantage. The fact that the iron it contains exists in the state of a protoxide is of considerable importance. As a general rule, in chalybeate waters the iron is usually found as a carbonate. It is generally conceded that sulphate chalybeate waters are greatly superior to carbonates. In the words of Dr Alexander, a well-known authority on the subject, 'they possess infinitely greater medical powers than the carbonate chalybeates'.

The University College of North Wales confirmed the above in its statement on the microbial origin of the Trefriw Wells Spa Water:

> The iron-rich mineral water that springs from Trefriw Wells owes its remarkable composition to the activity of bacteria living below ground in the mountainside. The process they carry out is entirely natural and the bacteria themselves are completely innocuous. They are remarkable, however, on two counts.
>
> Firstly, they possess a very high tolerance to acidic conditions — acidity is frequently used as a means of preservation against microbial spoilage, but these particular bacteria can live and thrive in extremely acidic environments, e.g. in dilute sulphuric acid, pH 1.5.
>
> Secondly, they are able to trap and utilise the chemical energy in certain mineral ores, most notably pyrite. The ore body embedded in the hillside is a particularly pure, fine-grain pyritous rock, which is of considerable age. The mineral pyrite contains two elements, iron and sulphur, in the form of FeS_2 (ferrous sulphide). It is a hard, dense material, and very stable in oxygen-depleted environments. However, in most aerated situations it changes form, or oxidises, to ferric sulphate. The process is slow abiotically, but in the presence of 'iron' and 'sulphur' bacteria is speeded up by about one million times.
>
> Both the iron and sulphur moieties change state, and these oxidation reactions release a little bit of energy which the specialised bacteria are able to utilise, in much the same way as green plants trap sunlight energy. Again, like green plants, they use carbon dioxide from the atmosphere to make a new

biomass (thus helping to counterbalance the 'greenhouse effect'). The oxidised forms of iron and sulphur are held in solution, due to the acidity also produced by the bacteria; in most situations the iron, in particular, would precipitate out, but the bacterial activity retains it, thus giving rise to the high concentration in the spring water. At the spring source itself, much of the iron is present as the reduced, ferrous form (due to chemical reactions occurring between the pyrite and ferric iron). It is this form which is more readily assimilated by the human body. The bacteria, known as *Thiobacillus ferro-oxidans*, *Thiobacillus thio-oxidans* and *Leptospitillum ferro-oxidans* have been studied by scientists for some years, and are being used increasingly in biotechnological operations.

Around 1925, Sir Humphry Rolleston wrote *The Spas of Great Britain*, subtitled *The official handbook of the British Spas Federation*. The publication of this interesting book included a foreword by the Committee for the Study of Medical Hydrology which reads as follows:

> The subject of medical hydrology, comprising the science of natural mineral waters and the art of their application, internally by drinking, and externally in the various forms of balneology, to the treatment of disease, is one for which little or no provision is made in the medical education, either graduate or post-graduate, in this country. The medical curriculum is so crowded that there is no room for a systematic course on the subject, and such knowledge as the student may gain is through an occasional lecture or demonstration, or is gradually acquired sporadically when, later on, he gets into practice. Nor is there any provision made for systematic post-graduate instruction. This state of affairs contrasts unfavourably with the position in certain foreign countries, notably France and Germany, where professorships or lectureships in Medical Hydrology are established in various universities.
>
> With a view to attempting to fill in the gap, a representative committee of medical men, practising in the British spas and in London, was formed in the year 1923.
>
> The matter was carefully inquired into, and the hope was entertained of creating a lectureship in Medical Hydrology

at the University of London. After consultation with the university authorities, the project was turned down, mainly on financial grounds, as it was found impossible to put up the amount necessary to endow a lectureship. As an alternative scheme, a panel of lecturers was formed, and the medical faculties of the universities of the United Kingdom and of the London Medical Schools were approached, and the offer made to them to provide lecturers, to be selected by them from the panel, to give a course of lectures each year on the subject of Medical Hydrology and Spa Treatment. It was clearly and definitely laid down by the promoters that the lectures would be purely educational and not tainted in any degree by matter that could be construed as advertisement of any particular spa, British or foreign. The lectures were to be followed by practical demonstrations, at one or other of the spas, of the balneological methods employed. The offer was accepted by most of the provincial universities, and lectures have been given annually at some, every two years at others, to fourth- and fifth-year students at the following universities: Belfast, Birmingham, Bristol, Dublin, Edinburgh, Glasgow, Leeds, Liverpool and Manchester. From reports received it would appear that the instruction given has proved of real value to the students.

A further development of the scheme has been the provision of lecturers to Medical Societies in various parts of the country, to branches of the British Medical Association, and to Post-graduate Institutions. These lectures are illustrated by films or lantern slides, so that those who cannot afford to visit a spa can have ocular demonstration of the methods employed.

The value of physical methods of treatment for many chronic diseases is being increasingly realised by the medical profession at large; and an insight into the indications for spa treatment, the methods employed, and the selection of a suitable spa, cannot fail to be of value to all engaged in medical practice.

An important part of the work of the committee is the arranging, from time to time, for parties of medical graduates and students to visit the home spas for practical demonstrations.

It seems to me that it is a great pity that these schemes are no longer available!

Most of my working life has been spent in Scotland and quite a few of my elderly patients have at some time or another expressed their regret that the Bridge of Allan Spa in the south of Scotland has been closed. Now they are equally delighted to learn that some of the once well-known spas have opened their doors again.

It is interesting to see that the waters of many of the spas possess different properties. I mentioned the Gasteiner Heilstollen in Austria in an earlier chapter. Gasteiner water has unique qualities. At this spa the minerals and trace elements are absorbed into the body through the skin in the hot baths and/or vapour baths. In the case of drinking cures, they are absorbed through the intestines, and in the tunnel cure, as well as in the vapour bath, cure through inhalation. Within the body, among other effects, its properties stimulate the various organic functions and promote internal glandular secretion, improve the circulation of the blood and act to regulate the blood pressure — as such, this water stabilises and regenerates the entire system.

We have also learned that the water at Lourdes, where millions of people find comfort and hope, contains the mineral germanium. This mineral is a vehicle for the release of oxygen in the body, hence the reason why people who are experiencing problems with their immunity receive a boost to their immune system. I always advise patients who inform me that they are going to Lourdes that they ought to drink as much of the water as possible while they are there.

We must realise that all the oxygen we require is obtainable from our food — from plants and animals, and from the fish in the sea that have fed on plankton and algae. Plankton is our greatest source of oxygen and it is therefore serious cause for concern when we see plankton rotting away because mankind is polluting its natural habitat with dangerous waste material. We seem to feel at liberty to dispose of anything unwanted in the world's seas and so encourage the destruction of creation.

Our modern dietary habits often seem to result in mineral deficiencies and this may be the reason why natural spa water can be so beneficial, as it can help to compensate for these deficiencies. There is no doubt that our planet is under attack from adverse atmospheric influences. At the creation of our planet clouds of hydrogen condensed under the force of gravity, creating intense pressure and releasing free energy. Of all the elements that were formed, only 92 had been identified until relatively recently; today the total is 103. Of these, the first 53 elements are concerned with life, i.e. our life depends on these in terms of structure and function. However, these minerals can only function when they are in a form that can be absorbed. This is what is meant when the 'ionic state' is mentioned, i.e. the mineral is available to us by virtue of its being in a soluble state and thus contained in the water. Unless the water concerned has been atmospherically affected, let us therefore drink as much of it as we can.

Minerals are nutrients that are necessary for the structure and function of all the cells in our bodies and we obtain them from our intake of food and fluids. Minerals in spa water have three major functions:

1. as constituents of all healthy cells of the body, i.e. bones, ligaments, muscles, blood and nerve cells;
2. as part of the body's biochemical make-up and physiological processes, i.e. they act as catalysts or metalo-enzymes in biological reactions such as muscle responses, the transmission of nerve impulses, digestion, absorption, the utilisation of other nutrients and hormone production;
3. as part of the mechanism for maintaining the delicate water- and acid-based balance in the body, which is essential for the proper functioning of all mental and physical processes by controlling the movements of nutrients

into, and waste products out of, the body cells. In this respect minerals are vital in the optimisation of all aspects of the body's defences against pollution, stress and infections because of their role in the immune system function.

Minerals, on the whole, are not stored in the body and need to be replenished daily; unlike other essential nutrients such as vitamins they cannot be manufactured. The primary sources of minerals are the soil and water. Unfortunately, the indiscriminate use of chemical fertilisers has led to the depletion of minerals available in the soil. In addition, the cultivation of plants for direct human consumption or as part of the human food chain is becoming affected by:

— the pressures of high levels of humic acid from acid rain, which results in minerals being made unavailable;
— the presence of other minerals, e.g. low levels of potassium or high levels of phosphates, fertilisers, pesticides or insoluble iron;
— the overall increase in acidity in many soils and the disturbance of the relationship between minerals within these soils.

As minerals can be considered as the lowest common denominator of disease and its prevention and cure — they are essential for health and vital in combatting disease — we must do all that lies within our power to protect their sources from pollution and other threats.

At this very moment, as I sit in the consulting room of my clinic, I can see the many people who are visiting the thermal baths in Arcen, to enjoy the water pumped up from a depth of nearly 900 metres, unaffected by interference from pesticides, insecticides and other chemicals. There are quite a few familiar faces among them, regulars who come back again and again to take the waters as it relieves them of their pain. I look beyond the clinic to the beautiful surroundings provided by nature and ask myself again why there is so much illness, disease and suffering in the world. I wonder how much of it is self-inflicted, and yet I also know the extent to which it is within our power to reverse the situation.

Many patients happily tell me about the considerable improvement they have noticed since they started to follow a multi-disciplinary programme and how they have benefited from the thermal mineral waters. The temperature of the water is a steady 34-35 °C (93-95 °F) and even in the coldest winters people who use it experience a reduction in pain. One gentleman whose neck and shoulders had stiffened considerably told me that it had become near enough impossible for him to continue driving his car, and even the most undemanding movements and tasks had become very troublesome. After having taken the cure in the thermal water he proudly boasted that he was now back to his old self. Because the pain had disappeared he was also able to sleep much better, but he was still puzzled by the fact that something so apparently innocuous as the water at Arcen can have such far-reaching effects.

Perhaps he would be less puzzled if he were to take into account the full extent of the water's rich mineral content. A research team from the Geochemistry Department of the University of Utrecht investigated the composition of the thermal water of Arcen and came up with the following results:

Cations (positively charged ions)	mg/litre
Natrium (Na)	10300.00
Lithium (Li)	10.10
Potassium (K)	295.00
Magnesium (Mg)	320.00
Calcium (Ca)	1040.00
Strontium (Sr)	52.00
Barium (Ba)	0.19
Manganese (Mn)	0.56

Anions (negatively charged ions)	mg/litre
Chloride (Cl)	18100.00
Sulphate (SO_4)	618.00
Bicarbonate (HCO_3)	903.00
Bromine (Br)	25.00
Phosphate (PO_4)	3.10
Iodine (I)	1.50
Fluoride (F)	1.80
Sulphide (S--)	0.08
Sulphide (HS--)	1.33
Carbon Dioxide (CO_2)	176.00

Was a visit to a spa merely considered an essential feature of their social calendar by our predecessors, or did they arrange these often elaborate visits in order to benefit physically? Or could it have been a combination of both factors? I would imagine that the answer to this would depend on the individual. However, because of the hidden dangers in today's environment, the health benefits to be gained from visiting a spa are possibly more important than ever before, as doing so can provide us with a measure of immunity to widespread pollutive influences. Therapeutically, a visit to a spa or thermal bath provides much more than an opportunity to relax or find relief from minor aches and pains. The curative and immunising properties of such waters can give us a new lease of life.

There is no doubt in the mind of Professor Izeng, of the Ludwig Maximilian University in Munich. He firmly believes that thermal mineral water is of the greatest benefit for rheumatism, arthritis, bowel complaints and heart and circulatory problems. No matter how deep we have had to drill to find this gift from nature, it is now greatly appreciated.

89

8

Water for Fitness

WHENEVER WE FEEL tired a nice hot bath will leave us feeling refreshed and relaxed at the same time. A cold bath may be even better, but unless one is used to cold baths they are usually a rather daunting prospect. To my mind, the best way of all is to have a hot shower and then briefly plunge into a cold tub. It is always a good idea to do this at the local swimming baths. Indeed, swimming is one of the finest all-round exercises for fitness that exists. It improves our general health and fitness, induces a pleasant, relaxed feeling and gives us a healthy appetite. As I have tried to point out so far in this book, a suitable water treatment exists for every mood or condition and it is certainly the case that water treatments can be adapted to enhance our general health and fitness.

When I am consulted by female patients about pre-menstrual tension, or menstrual or menopausal problems, I often suggest they take some form of water treatment. This will usually sort out their minor problems. If further help is needed we can take care of that in other ways, but in many cases no subsequent treatment will be required. A swollen stomach or bloated feeling during the premenstrual period or menstruation itself can be easily overcome by a regular swim, say two or three times a week. Swimming will also be helpful if there is undue pressure on the arteries. If it is inconvenient to visit the baths for a swim, take a long, cold sitz bath instead, again two or three times a week. I can assure you that doing so will ease your complaints.

The male menopause is now fully recognised by the medical profession, not merely as something that is all in the mind, but as a problem that expresses itself in physical ways as well, even though it may not be as marked as with the female menopause. I recently read a down-to-earth article on fathers who suffered from post-natal depression. This term is traditionally used to describe the feelings that many women experience shortly after giving birth. And now many men believe that they have also experienced the 'baby blues', saying that they felt empty or low, and were even prone to bursting into tears. Around 90 per cent of fathers now actively involve themselves in the birth of their children and the majority of these are believed to suffer from some form of depression in the postpartum period, i.e. the first few days after the birth. It must be stressed, however, that it would be wrong to suggest that men suffer from true post-natal depression. This term can be used to describe a condition which can vary markedly in terms of duration and severity. Where fathers are concerned, suffering from 'post-natal blues' largely involves a period of brief and mild fluctuations of the emotions and this is not regarded as an illness. In mothers, however, various, much more serious and longer-term forms of depression can occur.

I have strayed from the subject, however. The male menopause can cause a variety of problems, both mental and physical, which can prey heavily on middle-aged males. Like the advice for females during the menopause, here again I would suggest a regular swim or cold sitz bath for the males.

Elderly men who experience problems when urinating would be well advised to take frequent hot baths to which some *Solidago* (goldenrod) or chamomile has been added. Even sitting on the edge of a hot bath containing an infusion of these herbs will be of help, as long as the hot vapours from the bath can reach the lower part of the body and so assist in stimulating the urinating function.

Chronic constipation doubtlessly affects a person's fitness. This is not the first time that I have stressed the importance of regular bowel movements, and those people with a tendency to constipation should remember to drink plenty of fluids. It is also helpful to take some active form of water treatment, such as swimming, or to take a cold sitz bath or perform dry brush massages.

The well-known Schlenz cure is of great importance for those who wish to improve their physical fitness. You may be surprised to learn that the Schlenz method was not developed by a physician or naturopath, but by a housewife and mother. She had used the water therapies advocated by Father Kneipp and instinctively recognised the significance of these methods for overall health. Along with the cold-water treatment, this particular form of hydrotherapy is widely recognised by doctors as being effective and is often recommended. The general recommendation is that the Schlenz method is adopted once or twice a week, although in Eastern countries it tends to be done on a more frequent basis. Some practitioners advise that the temperature of the bath water is raised to two or three degrees above blood temperature. However, if the temperature is raised by 4-5 degrees to 41 or 42 °C (105.8-107.6 °F), the blood will circulate more quickly and is more likely to effect an improvement in certain swellings that may have formed in the body. It is claimed that this treatment is of particular benefit in the treatment of tumours. However, if you decide to try this method, it is important that you first familiarise yourself with all aspects of it.

Firstly, the tub used for a Schlenz bath needs to be longer than a normal bath, and if at all possible it should be constructed from wood. When taking a Schlenz bath the head should always be kept above the water level, and some thought should be given to devising a method to safeguard the patient from slipping down in the bath. The position adopted must allow the patient to breathe easily through both the mouth and the nose. At the start, the temperature of the bath water should be about 36-37 °C (96.8-98.6 °F, or blood temperature); this is then raised by the addition of hot water to 38 °C (100.4 °F). It must be remembered that the temperature of the water should not be allowed to go down; it is better that it is increased slightly. During this treatment it is considered important to drink some herbal tea, or a few drops of Dr Vogel's Crataegisan dissolved in some water.

Dr Vogel, who has studied this method carefully, is strongly in favour of this form of water therapy and has advised many of his patients accordingly. Dr Vogel is also a great believer in the wisdom of Parmenides, who, as I have noted before, said: 'Give me the power to raise the temperature and I will heal every illness.' A greater degree of heat can indeed be a healing factor and if the temperature of the water is finally raised to 40 or 41 °C (105.6-107.6 °F), the sensitive pathogens can be destroyed. Not only is this method effective in the treatment of viruses and indeed tumour cells, it is also of great help to the blood circulation and beneficial to the lymphatic system.

In the early stages, a Schlenz bath should never take longer than half an hour. As time goes on, this may be increased by anything up to two hours. In cases of obesity it is useful to add some sea salt to the bath water, or even to use sea water. After the bath the patient should take care to sit for a while to allow the body temperature to regulate itself and this is done by sitting quietly, covered by hot woollen blankets, until the body has cooled down. To encourage this process, dab a little PoHo oil under the nose or concentrate on regular breathing. A little St John's wort oil could be gently rubbed into the skin while the skin is still warm and this will increase the feeling of general well-being.

In many cases, the person who has just taken a Schlenz bath feels so relaxed that all he or she wants to do is retire to bed. For this reason it would be ideal if this method could be followed at home. Although the treatment could easily be obtained in a sauna or Turkish bath, the benefits of having this facility at home should not be underestimated. It need not be too expensive to install suitable equipment at home and it is more likely that the benefits would far outweigh the initial investment.

Patients with multiple sclerosis and hormonal imbalances have found great benefit from the Schlenz method and for that reason alone it deserves recognition.

Arthritic people, who often feel tired because of the constant pain, will also benefit from this method, as they will from most forms of hydrotherapy. They will also gain relief from alternate cold and hot showers, as well as alternate cold and hot compresses applied locally. I can heartily recommend a sauna or a Turkish bath to such patients, and also baths to which Epsom salts or bicarbonate of soda have been added. Seaweed baths, sea-water baths and moderate sunbathing are all helpful for arthritic conditions. Hot and cold compresses with some castor oil applied to specific painful areas can also be soothing.

Asthma and bronchitis patients should combine the Schlenz bath with hot foot baths.

Emphysema patients are advised to bathe their wrists in hot water containing Epsom salts. The use of hot fermentations with PoHo oil will also give great relief.

Psoriasis is a difficult condition to get under control and much effort may be required. In my book *Arthritis, Rheumatism and Psoriasis* I have given very specific advice for such patients, and I have already mentioned the marvellous results to be obtained from the mineral salts found in the Dead Sea, but additional water treatment is very important. Please remember that psoriasis cannot be cured from the outside, and therefore the dietary advice provided in the book named above will be of great help to those who suffer from this complaint. In addition, swim and sunbathe as often as possible. Sun treatment after swimming has proved to be of considerable benefit. Also, care of the colon is important, which is why I always advise that herbal tea is taken regularly. I must stress, however, that one of the best treatments for psoriasis that exists is a swim in the sea followed by some sunbathing.

Colitis and diverticulitis are becoming increasingly common, and it is important that these conditions are recognised in their early stages and to know what dietary measures should be taken. Cold compresses applied over the abdomen will reduce inflammation and, as colon irritation is an important factor in these conditions, colonics, or hot herbal concoctions, are usually found helpful by such patients.

A naturopath may make a considerable effort to either increase or lower a fever. A high fever may exceed 40 °C (104 °F) and this serves as an indication of the severity of the problem. The duration of such a fever is also an important factor, and therefore whenever a rise in temperature is suspected it must be measured correctly, because the physician will need such information to guide him in his diagnosis. It is significant that when animals are ill they refuse to eat and, as their actions are very much ruled by their instincts, we may deduce that this is how nature intended it to be. However, give the feverish patient plenty of liquids, whether it be water, diluted fruit juices or hot herbal teas. Other forms of water treatment to bring down a fever may include cold compresses placed over the stomach, hot blanket baths, hot Epsom salts baths, bicarbonate of soda baths, or a normal bath followed by an extensive body rub.

Haemorrhoids and varicose veins are both circulatory problems and here, too, water treatments will be helpful. As always, prevention is better than cure and in this context also, water treatments can be applicable. For pain relief use hot compresses and hot sitz baths. Later, hot and cold sitz baths can be taken or, as an alternative, hot and cold compresses. For acute cases, ice-packs and cold compresses with some St John's wort oil or *Hamamelis* extract, sometimes alternated with lemon juice compresses, may help to relieve these uncomfortable conditions.

Migraines and headaches can be eased by placing an ice-cold compress at the base of the head while lying in a darkened room. An even more effective treatment is to place an ice-pack on the forehead while taking a hot foot bath at the same time. Continue this treatment for 10-15 minutes while relaxing in a prone position and in most cases the headache or migraine will disappear spontaneously.

Over the years, I have been asked to treat an unusually large number of multiple sclerosis patients at my clinics and here, more than with any other condition, I believe that an acceptable level of general fitness is of the utmost importance. Most of the water treatments I have described in this book are suitable for multiple sclerosis patients, but it should always be remembered that although bathing in either the sea or a swimming pool is allowed, multiple sclerosis patients should never sunbathe afterwards. There appears to be some controversy on this subject, but in my experience direct sunshine is detrimental to such patients. Exercise out of doors is excellent and daily alternate hot and cold showers are definitely recommended, but please, no sunbathing. When spending time out of doors, lie down and relax in a shady position and breathe in the fresh air, but always try to stay out of the immediate rays of strong sunlight.

On the subject of general fitness I would like to emphasise the need to care for our kidneys. The kidneys may be likened to the laboratory of our whole system and with due care and attention they will work unstintingly for our benefit. A number of water treatments are beneficial for the kidneys, but none more so than drinking an ample daily quantity of good-quality drinking water, which will flush out the kidneys and help them to dispose of toxins in a natural way. Bathing in the sea is also helpful and if the kidneys appear to be overworked, you can also place hot and cold compresses on that area of the stomach. A final point to remember is to always be sparing in the use of kitchen salt.

Water for fitness — so much can be said about it. What is required is mostly a matter of common sense. Using the above guidelines to set you on the right road, you will soon be able to adapt some of the treatments I have described to suit your specific needs and circumstances. There is really nothing new about hydrotherapy; I have already explained that the therapeutic value of hydrotherapy has been acknowledged for many centuries. Please note that the therapeutic effects will vary according to the electric fields of certain waters and their content of minerals and trace elements. The latter will vary according to the source of the water, and whether it is filtered through lime, clay or peat layers. All these circumstances will determine the eventual healing factor.

9

Water Pollutants

ALTHOUGH I HAVE already referred to many pollutants, by no means have all of them been mentioned (see the map opposite). This must be done in order to enable you to recognise these substances as constituting a danger to your general health and that of your family. For the sake of specific threats to the immune system and the alarming increase of allergic reactions we encounter today, this particular problem must be thoroughly investigated.

Let us consider first the nitrate problem. Once inside the body nitrates combine with amines, which are present in most foods, to form nitrosamines, which are highly carcinogenic compounds. Many of the British water authorities currently lack the appropriate purification equipment and it is believed that millions of people in Britain are consuming water that contains nitrates at a level which is above the EEC limits. In quite a few areas, and specifically that around the Thames, the nitrate level in the water is cause for considerable concern, as many of the nitrates originate from agricultural fertilisers that have filtered into the water

98

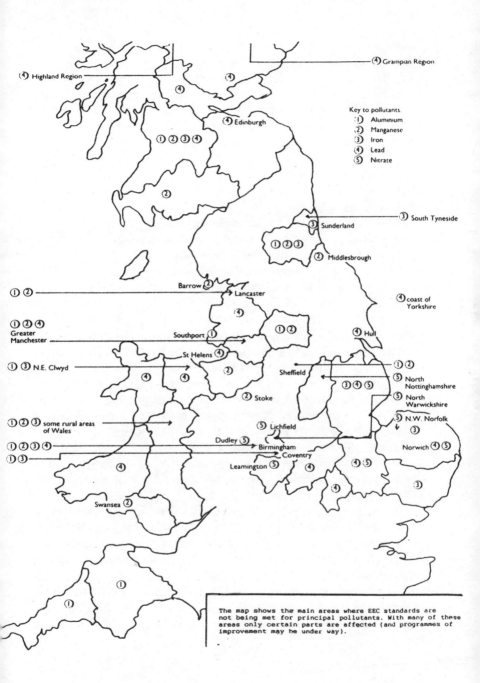

④ Grampian Region

④ Highland Region

④

④

④ Edinburgh

Key to pollutants:
① Aluminium
② Manganese
③ Iron
④ Lead
⑤ Nitrate

① ② ③ ④

②

③ Sunderland   ③ South Tyneside

① ② ③

② Middlesbrough

① ②   ② Barrow

Lancaster

④   ④ coast of Yorkshire

④
Greater Manchester   Southport ①

① ②   ④ Hull

① ③ N.E. Clwyd   St Helens ④

④   ④   ②

① ②

Sheffield   ① ②

③ ④ ⑤   ⑤ North Nottinghamshire

② Stoke   ⑤ North Warwickshire

① ② ③ some rural areas of Wales

⑤ Lichfield   ⑤ N.W. Norfolk

① ② ③ ④   Dudley ⑤

① ③   Birmingham   Norwich ④ ⑤

Coventry

④   Leamington ⑤   ④   ④ ⑤

②

④   ③

Swansea ②

①

①

The map shows the main areas where EEC standards are not being met for principal pollutants. With many of these areas only certain parts are affected (and programmes of improvement may be under way).

table. Considering modern farming methods, this presents a very grim picture because there does not seem to be an easy solution to this problem. In agricultural terms, the nitrates that have been added to the soil will reappear in vegetation and, subsequently, through the food chain in meat, especially pork, as well as in the water supplies. The extent to which our meat supply has been contaminated with nitrates and other toxins has become a great worry, and is a subject that has received a considerable amount of publicity recently, which has intensified as a result of the controversy surrounding BSE ('Mad Cow Disease'). We would all be well advised to supplement our diet with vitamin C to protect ourselves against the influence of nitrates and nitrites and make our immune system as effective as possible.

In the *Sunday Times* of 3 July 1988, there appeared an article on how the British authorities were planning to spend millions of pounds to safeguard the quality of our drinking water and ward against carcinogenic influences entering our water supplies. To my way of thinking, the only sensible approach to achieving this aim must be to start at the source, rather than adding non-essential chemicals to the water at a later stage. I am greatly concerned that by restricting any action to the latter, this is merely a case of adding insult to injury. For example, in an effort to reduce dental decay among the population, and most specifically among the younger generation, the authorities — in their wisdom — have given permission for the addition of fluoride to the public water supplies, i.e. a compound with carcinogenic characteristics.

In another newspaper report, this time in *The Observer* of Sunday, 12 June 1988, a link between polluted water and dementia was made and it was claimed, and it continues to be claimed, that water pollutants are of great concern in connection with Alzheimer's disease. The water authorities are embarrassed about such claims and do not know how to react to them; nevertheless, it is clearly the case that the risk of disease increases in line with the level of metals in the drinking water. This has been shown where the EEC limit of 200 micrograms of aluminium per litre of drinking water has been exceeded, suggesting that our current limits are too lax. Certainly, of all the possible pollutants, aluminium contamination presents us with the most serious threats. A book written by Dr Peter Mansfield together with his co-author, Dr Jean Monro, entitled *Chemical Children — How to Protect Your Family from Harmful Pollution*, outlines the dangers and will be of great interest to anyone who is concerned about the possible effects of polluted drinking water. The potential links between aluminium and Alzheimer's disease are discussed further in later pages.

The pollution of our waterways by nitrogen is definitely an ever-increasing problem but it need not necessarily be insurmountable. It is not only the chemical fertilisers that are responsible for nitrogen pollution; other artificial chemicals used in the manufacture of pesticides and insecticides must also share the blame. The simplest solution here would be to turn the clock back and re-establish the old method of recycling farmyard manure and spreading it over the fields as a fertiliser. Let the farmers also plough the straw back into the soil during the autumn and then the bacteria can set to work on breaking down some of the nitrogen it contains — and we would all live in a safer environment. Research has shown that in order to reduce the amount of pollution it would help if we all tried to think more along the lines of organic farming; even if it were only in our own gardens to start with, we might all be pleasantly surprised at how good the yield would be.

I was intrigued to read an article about a trust in Wales where 43,000 acres of unspoilt land in the Elan Valley were leased with an endowment of £100,000. The objectives of the trust are to preserve, maintain and enhance the area and its animal and plant life, to encourage public access, to promote a study of the area and its wildlife and to encourage use of the Elan Valley for charitable purposes. The lease contains certain restrictions, among the most

101

WATER

important of which are those protecting the flow of water into the reservoirs and preventing commercial development being undertaken by the trustees. This indeed offers an ideal opportunity to show what can be achieved in organic farming and, hopefully, some lessons will be learned from this experiment that can be applied on a larger scale.

Water always did, and still should, have nutritional value, and especially in the conditions described above it could well hold the balance as a decisive factor in the project's success. According to Dr Stephen Davis, the chairperson of the British Society of Nutritional Medicine, tap water is a vital dietary supplement. The essential mineral elements we should get from it, he says, ought to include calcium, magnesium, zinc and iodine, among many others.

There is a very high prevalence of zinc deficiency in Britain, and I often recognise this condition in my patients. When a supplement of zinc is then added to their diet we often achieve surprising results. Similar results are also obtained after using the Trefriw Wells mineral water, which has a high content of natural iodine, and is extremely beneficial. Nutrition from food, of which water is such an essential part, is also of great relevance in correcting deficiencies that affect human mental development.

Certain household purification methods deserve much greater attention as it is not unknown for the reverse osmosis process to destroy many health-giving properties in the water. In some cases the removal of essential minerals can even make the water more toxic than before it was filtered. You will surely realise why I am so insistent that this subject continues to be studied in depth, in order to provide us with a healthier environment — for everyone's benefit.

We owe it to ourselves and to future generations to work very hard to ensure that our drinking water does not contain any substances that may adversely affect our health. We must bring pressure to bear on the national and local authorities to make sure that our water is safe to drink, and that it does not in any way constitute a risk to human health. In this effort it is of little use or comfort to learn that various components are added or extracted from the water which is vital to the survival of mankind.

During a visit to the United States I was taken on a tour of a food-processing factory. I was greatly concerned when I learned about the process of injecting water into various foods and the dangers this presents from the point of view of bacteria being introduced. I saw that chickens and turkeys, for example, were injected with water to increase their weight before being sold. In some cases, this leads to proteins being made more soluble, thereby encouraging water retention, and only a percentage of this injected water is lost during the cooking process. All these aspects can endanger our health. Processed food manufacturers claim that polyphosphates increase the succulence and juiciness of the finished product. However, consumers must decide for themselves whether the resulting sogginess is what is required. British manufacturers are not bound by any maximum limits with regard to water content in the preparation of processed foods, which I find extremely worrying. Polyphosphates are also added to the brine that is injected into carcass meat and forms part of the meat-moulding process. It is also the case that the extra weight must be paid for by the customer, and in this way the price of meat is kept artificially high. Recent research has indicated some added dangers, as polyphosphates have been found to act as blocking agents against certain enzymes in the human body and can thus cause digestive problems. The overall picture is most disturbing, and the discovery of 'Mad Cow Disease' should not come as a great surprise when we consider that cattle are bombarded with chemical fertilisers, growth hormones, antibiotics, tranquillisers and pesticides.

In one report I read that the amount of water injected into meat can often be quite staggering; for example, a joint of bacon with a declared water content of 15 per cent may actually contain up to 24 per cent water — with the surplus being matched by other additives. A frozen product may be ice-glazed, while the real, defrosted weight is much less than that stated on the label. Convenience foods as a whole have a substantially higher water content than do fresh foods. This must surely give us food for thought!

Let us not lose sight of the fact that water pollutants are present in our domestic cleaning materials and detergents. Water in itself ought to be considered as a cleanser, but we then add chemical detergents to the water we use for washing and cleaning, and all of these additives have to end up somewhere, namely, in our rivers and oceans. The microbes — small bacteria — which are necessary for the water's own 'housekeeping' are often killed by such substances and the various water animals and plants will begin to die off. The great West European river, the Rhine, is now so badly polluted that there is hardly any plant growth or fish life left and swimming in its water is largely forbidden, in some places by law. We appear to just accept all these developments and it makes me wonder if we are ever going to stand up for ourselves and do something about them. How are we going to force the establishment to take note of public concern? Some manufacturers have already paid heed, fortunately, and indeed already there are several brands of phosphate-free washing powder available which represent a reduced health risk. If we listen to our conscience we should all consider supporting this drive, as we are also obliged to do in relation to the lead-free petrol option.

From statistics it would appear that in the Netherlands 40,000 tonnes of phosphates are being dumped into the country's inland waters: 40 per cent from industrial sources, 22 per cent from human faeces, 21 per cent from detergents, 13 per cent from artificial manure and 4 per cent from various unidentified sources. If we think how little consideration we pay to whether we keep the tap running or not, we all know deep down that we could easily be more economical with the use of our tap water, and in this way we will be accepting a certain amount of responsibility for the conservation of this natural resource. An average bath takes 125 litres of water, while an average shower consumes only 50 litres. How often do we notice that a tap has not been turned off properly and unless it is pointed out to us, we will probably continue to be careless in this respect unless we are charged for our water according to the amount used in our individual households. Only then will we consider having our dripping taps repaired. Remember, sensible water conservation can only help in our efforts to effect a reduction in water pollutants. If we can reduce the quantity of water used, I am sure that we can coincidentally improve the quality of the water. Water is fast becoming a valuable asset and as such it deserves to be treated with respect.

Today, there is more acceptance of the belief that our immune systems would be in better shape if there were fewer water pollutants, because viruses would not be able to get such an easy hold on our system. The so-called chronic fatigue syndrome (ME, or post-viral syndrome) is making strident increases and this would not be the case if our water was not affected by so many pollutants — and this is only a single example. In this context I am reminded of the elderly farmer and his wife who presented me with such clear evidence of having fallen prey to such adverse conditions (see page 14). My findings in that particular case were borne out by a more detailed study which later took place in that area, and in the future more studies of toxic processes will have to be undertaken to either confirm or rule out whether a number of cases of illness have been caused by certain substances, as was the case with the elderly couple who came to me for treatment.

In a report prepared by one of the Glasgow hospitals it is stated quite clearly that there is great concern as to the possible connections between the rural environment and the chronic fatigue syndrome. Thinking back to the early days when I was consulted by people who were diagnosed eventually as suffering from ME, I came to realise that they all were residents of certain areas. At that time I would have been able to pinpoint on a map where clusters of patients hailed from. In view of the knowledge we have gained since those early days I consider it very likely that these areas could well have been affected by the disposal of waste or other toxic material, and therefore I am a firm believer that polluted water must be considered as being detrimental to the immune system.

How are we going to clean up these pollutants? Surely not by adding further chemicals to the water, and least of all by adding chemicals that are supposedly added for our 'protection'? Some years ago, I wrote to the Secretary of State for Health in relation to the government's fluoridation plans, suggesting that we did not want massive self-medication. Also on this big question of fluoridation I asked the government representative why it was not considered necessary to go the whole way and also add some laxatives to the water while they were about it, because, after all, half the population seems to experience constipation problems! We should all be aware that it is within our democratic rights to refuse the addition of certain supposed 'self-medication' products to our water, as certain products are used of which we do not have sufficient knowledge and it has not been proved conclusively that they will not cause harmful side-effects.

In the excellent book *Fluoride — The Freedom Fight*, by my good friend Dr Hans Moolenburgh, we can read about the dangers of fluoridation and also about the tremendous controversies in which he became personally involved when he dared to voice his objections to a fluoridation programme proposed by Dutch authorities. He was joined initially by only a handful of dissenters, but their efforts to point out to the establishment the dangers inherent in the addition of fluoride to the public water supply eventually gained huge popular support. The dissenters organised themselves into a powerful lobby and at long last won their battle and managed to prevent the implementation of the programme. I would like to believe that common sense will eventually prevail everywhere. Too many tests have left enough grounds for suspicion that fluoride can be harmful. In Britain we have been less successful in this battle to convince the government bodies responsible for this decision that without all the relevant background information this regulation should not be enforced. Many more in-depth studies will be required before we fully understand the consequences of adding this chemical to the public water supplies.

I remember a certain patient whose condition caused me great concern, while I could not find any plausible reason for her ill health. In due course I realised that it was an allergic reaction to some pollutant in the water. It took a great amount of care and effort to turn the tide, but at long last we managed to undo most of the harm that had affected her, although she had been suffering from a multitude of severe problems.

Despite their valiant efforts, the National Pure Water Association lost the battle against the deliberate pollution of our public water supplies and the British fluoridation programme went ahead. This Association's aim was to promote the protection of the public water supplies from *all* forms of contamination. They felt compelled to oppose the views of the relevant government bodies in the supply of mass medication through these unusual channels. They are still active in their battle and, fortunately, though only slowly, they are now receiving some credit for their efforts; hopefully, common sense will prevail in the end.

In the latest newsletter issued by the National Pure Water Association I read that as far as fluoridation in the United

107

States is concerned, and by implication in the other countries worldwide with fluoridation schemes, it will be the Environmental Protection Agency (EPA) which will make the final decision about whether or not to allow the addition of fluoride to drinking water to continue (at present the EPA standard, set in 1985, allows a maximum of 4 ppm fluoride).

It is believed that the EPA will come under strong political and economic pressure *not* to declare fluoride a carcinogen and thus prohibit its presence as an addition to drinking water. Many US public water supplies contain relatively high levels of fluoride — which would have to be removed at considerable expense. The artificial fluoridation lobby would also suffer a loss of 'face'. The manufacturers — mainly the phosphate fertiliser industries — would lose a profitable outlet for this waste; moreover, these industries could come under pressure from the international 'green' movement because the waste fluorides that are currently extracted from the waste gases will once again be discharged into the atmosphere, resulting in environmental damage and claims from farmers and others caused by this damaging form of air pollution.

Nevertheless, there are strong reasons to believe that fluoride is harmful. From a report compiled in the United States following research into adverse health effects ascribed to fluoridation, I quote:

> The teeth of both rats and mice showed dental fluorosis symptoms during the two-year study. Malformation of the dentine layer, degeneration of ameloblasts and to a lesser extent of the odontoblast was observed, especially in rats. There was an increased incidence and severity of osteosclerosis in high-dose female rats but not in dosed male rats or mice.
>
> The incidence of liver neoplasms in all groups of dosed and controlled male and female mice was higher than has typically been seen in NTP studies. A review of pathology information from NTP studies which began about the same time as the sodium fluoride studies, but which has not yet

been completely evaluated and reported, has revealed a sharp increase in liver neoplasms, especially in females.

Again, I will quote from an article in the National Pure Water Association's newsletter:

In response to our enquiries about chemical impurities found in the fluorides used in water fluoridation, a number of specifications have been received, all identical. Apparently the Department of the Environment has laid down maximum acceptable levels for several chemical impurities which, when diluted, are insignificant compared to some chemical and other pollutants flowing from many taps in the British Isles.

A typical specification starts with:

'The product shall be colourless, free from suspended matter and must not contain any mineral or organic substances capable of impairing the health of those drinking water correctly treated with the product.'

The logical conclusion to be drawn from the above is that the product is unfit and the water industry should discontinue all fluoridation schemes because fluoride *will* impair the health of many water consumers, some of whom will develop cancer as a direct result of drinking fluoridated water.

Turning now to aluminium, a study by scientists from the Medical Research Council's Epidemiology Unit, its Neuro-chemical Pathology Unit and the Water Research Centre, shows a geographical relationship between Alzheimer's disease and aluminium in drinking water (*Lancet*, 14 January 1989).

In districts with a mean aluminium concentration greater than 0.01 mg per litre, the risk in patients under the age of seventy years of contracting Alzheimer's disease was 50 per cent higher than in districts where concentrations were less than 0.01 mg per litre. A further analysis of a sub-group of patients under the age of sixty-five years showed an even closer relation between aluminium concentration and Alzheimer's disease than in patients under the age of seventy years.

This survey was conducted in eighty-eight county districts within England and Wales. There was a greater than 50 per cent increase in dementia in the age group 40-65 in areas in the North East of England, the South West and North Wales, as compared to the rest of England and Wales.

It was understood that the effect of fluoride was also to have been examined in this study, but this was omitted, apparently for political reasons because of the impending privatisation of the water authorities.

Aluminium in drinking water only forms a small part (about 10 per cent) of the total intake, but because the aluminium is in a form which is easily assimilated it adds disproportionately to the total amount absorbed by the body.

The results of a French study, published in the Proceedings of the US National Academy of Science, December 1988, show the effect of a fluoride-aluminium chemical complex on the biochemistry of cells. Other recent research, conducted by a team led by Dr S. Norton at the University of Maine, also suggests the extreme toxicity of aluminium combined with fluorine following studies in fish biology. The levels at which cytotoxic effects were observed in fish and human cells is similar to the levels of alum flocculation used by certain British water authorities which also add fluoride to their supplies. It is clearly essential that epidemiological research is carried out as a matter of urgency and that fluoridation is discontinued immediately. This applies in particular in those areas where tap water supplies contain 0.02 mg per litre or more aluminium.

The EEC Guide Level (GL) for aluminium is 0.05 mg per litre and the Maximum Admissible Concentration (MAC) is 0.20 mg per litre. It appears essential for the sake of water consumers' health that these levels are drastically reduced without delay, pending the total abolition of aluminium in water purification processes.

The arguments put forward in favour of the use of aluminium are that this is the only method that works for the type of water in which it is used. But other safe methods *are* available at a higher cost. In addition, the water industry will suffer the loss of 'face' if aluminium is withdrawn from general use, not to mention the possibility of future legal action for damages on the part of affected water consumers. The Department of Health appears unwilling to publish the available statistics and does not appear to be prepared to provide funding for further detailed studies.

Most of us are aware of the damage caused by acid rain 'exported' from Britain and industrialised Europe to Norway and Sweden. In Norway, a geographical association has been found between aluminium levels in drinking water (deposited from acid rain) and dementia.

Some studies have been carried out in the British uplands where industrial acid deposits have been found to have caused damage to vegetation, birds and fish. Emissions from large industrial complexes increase the leaching of aluminium, zinc, lead, cadmium and other heavy metals into water courses and drinking water supplies. Consequently, many raw water supplies — the rivers, lakes and reservoirs from which the water authorities extract their water for further treatment and purification — contain high levels of aluminium and heavy metals.

A team of scientists from the University of Surrey conducted analyses of more than 900 water samples collected by members of the public during 1987/8. It was found that most elemental drinking water concentrations of heavy metals were below the EEC directive's guidelines, with the exceptions of aluminium and lead.

The National Osteoporosis Society has consistently promoted the use of fluoride in the treatment of osteoporosis. Consequently, many elderly women support fluoridation in the mistaken belief that this additional source of fluoride will help in the prevention of hip fractures.

The chairperson of the National Osteoporosis Society recently cited as 'the most compelling evidence for fluoride in the prevention of osteoporosis-related hip fractures' a paper presented by Simonen and Laitinen and published in *The Lancet* in 1985. On the basis of this paper he feels justified in continuing to uphold the conviction that fluoride is helpful in the prevention of osteoporosis.

This study by Simonen and Laitinen is a small, poorly-done study filled with errors that somehow escaped proper review before its publication in *The Lancet*. The authors collected their cases from a computer read-out of admissions to the hospitals of two Finnish towns, one fluoridated and one not. They did not realise that their technique was faulty since the sex-ratio incidence from the fluoridated town showed an equal ratio of men to women, when it is well established that the true ratio is 3-4 women to 1 man. In addition, they made several other errors and ignored another orthopaedic research paper published by the University of Kuopio, the fluoridated town of their flawed paper. The truth of the matter is that fluoride is toxic to bones at all levels tested and there is no benefit in relation to the prevention of osteoporosis.

The British Fluoridation Society has also claimed the benefits of fluoridation in the prevention of osteoporosis from time to time, apparently in order to boost its claims about 'additional' benefits to be gained from fluoridation.

An article that appeared in *The Journal* (Newcastle upon Tyne) of 20 July 1990 reads as follows:

> *Fluoride plans for a million people in the North*
> Moves to add fluoride to the water supplies of another one million consumers in the North-East have come a step closer following months of delay caused by legal worries.
> Northumbrian Water has agreed to add fluoride to its supplies after satisfying itself with the terms of a Government

decision to indemnify water companies from risk of damages claimed by consumers.

The company has had talks with the Northern Regional Health Authority but said yesterday it will fluoridate supplies when the RHA asks it to.

The Health Authority's current policy is that water supplies to all the region should be fluoridated in a bid to improve dental health.

Health authorities and dental experts in the region pressed for fluoridation for years, claiming it is the most cost-effective way to tackle tooth decay.

Earlier this year they attacked the delay as deplorable as it stood in the way of improving dental health. But many others believe there are other health risks with putting fluoride in water supplies.

Northumbrian Water, and other former water authorities, refused to fluoridate supplies until the Government promised to indemnify them against possible claims from customers who believe their health has been adversely affected by fluoridation.

The indemnity was granted almost a year ago and since then the water authorities have been studying implications before making a decision.

I have been quoted as saying that water is more important than food. To stay alive, water is essential — and the regeneration of water is therefore most important in today's world despite our technological achievements. Things have not changed that drastically and it is still true that prevention is better than cure. Considering the many illnesses, diseases and problems that can occur as a result of water pollution, it is time to take action. The evidence obtained in relation to the current water environment and technology speaks for itself. The development of certain treatment methods has helped to moderate pollution effects but the discovery of other assets has had a detrimental influence on what might have been achieved. The value of water and its quality deserves very serious consideration at any time, but never more so than today.

On a recent visit to Canada I became greatly concerned when I was informed about issues pertaining to the severe problems being experienced as a result of the pollution of the country's large bodies of water. Acknowledgement of these problems ought to go hand in hand with acceptance of the responsibility of their solution, for unless something is done very soon, it will be too late. No longer can we stand by and tolerate the abuse of one of nature's gifts so that it has a detrimental effect on human health.

> If a man can convince me and bring home to me that I do not think or act right, gladly will I change; for I search after truth, by which no man yet was harmed. But he is harmed who abideth on still in his deception and ignorance.
>
> (Marcus Aurelius)

10

Water of the Seas

ON A BUSY Saturday morning in the clinic my receptionist asked me if I was prepared to take an important telephone call. I found myself speaking to a professor, who explained that he held a chair at one of our well-known universities. He asked me if it was at all possible to meet him at a certain place because he had something very important to show me. I explained how busy I was and that my waiting-room was filled with patients waiting to see me and told him that it was impossible for me to come out straight away. He then said that he had discovered something that morning while taking his dog for a walk along the beach and assured me that I would be interested. He would not tell me what it was all about, but left me in no doubt that I would be equally fascinated by what he had to show me. I then agreed to meet him during the break I had allowed in my appointment system in the middle of the day.

When I arrived at our prearranged meeting place he pointed at some seaweed that was lying at the water's edge. It resembled a glowing and phosphorous mass of

115

tangles. It was clear that this seaweed had been washed ashore during the previous tide because it was still fresh and had not been washed high up onto the beach. In its own way it looked most impressive and in an odd way it had a beauty of its own. At the same time, the professor expressed great concern as to what the reason for its phosphorous luminosity might be. We discussed some of the possibilities and then we gathered some of the seaweed and took it away from the beach. The professor promised to have it analysed at the university laboratory. When the test results came through we were both staggered to say the least: the seaweed contained an incredibly high level of contamination and toxicity and it was unbelievable that this had only just been deposited onto the beach by the tide.

Later on, during the evening of that same day, when the clinic was closed, I decided to take another stroll to the beach. I had since had time to consider some of the possibilities and I have to admit that I was as intrigued as my learned friend. I stood in wonder and amazement as I considered how nature protects us from our present environment. For many years I have advocated that some of my patients take Kelpasan for various complaints. Kelpasan is a derivative of kelp (as the name indicates) and is marketed in the Bioforce range. It is made from pure sea algae from the Pacific Ocean and contains all their original trace elements. It serves as a natural supplement for iodine deficiencies and a prophylactic for goitre, and it stimulates the cell metabolism of the endocrine glands. It also increases mental and physical capacity.

Standing there on the shore, looking out over the Atlantic Ocean, I mused on the fact that here was visible proof that the seaweed at my feet had absorbed some of the rubbish that mankind had seen fit to dispose of by dumping it into the sea. In nature's own way, the seaweed had attracted these pollutants in an effort to minimise the detrimental effects it would have on the marine biology. It was an awesome moment when the realisation first dawned that nature had attempted to protect us from our own contamination of such natural resources and that the sea, in an attempt to refuse such abuse, had brought it back ashore to us. At the same time, it is a frightening thought if we consider that plankton, which to a large extent is responsible for our oxygen supply, is rotting away in some of the world's seas as a consequence of our negligence, ignorance and — even worse — our stupidity.

If we stop to think how helpful the sea can be in healing our bodies, how good a purpose it serves for our recreation and, ultimately, how it is such a tremendous source of life not only in terms of marine biology, we cannot fail to recognise that we ought to respect it much more than we do at present.

A little while ago I read a book called *Troubled Water*, by David Kinnersley. I have to admit that the contents of this book gave me a lot of food for thought and it reminded me of how negligent we are of our seas and rivers. I am sure the writer will forgive me if I share a worthwhile thought with you which he used to close one of his chapters dealing with the subject of water in nature and its political connections:

> Over the last century or so we have experienced revolution in so far that this natural resource is available to us on a lavish scale at a very minimal cost. We all enjoy the comfort of having water on tap for our everyday purposes, at home and at work. While this progress was going on we have all but forgotten about the essential endless renewal of this natural resource. In the late twentieth century we are learning that we are not dealing with an unlimited supply and to safeguard our future we cannot anymore leave its care to the experts. As involuntary neighbours in conventional sharing of water, especially in routine matters, we have to gain a fuller understanding of how our individual actions affect others.

These are wise words indeed by the author of this excellent book; indeed, throughout the whole of the book there are lessons to be learned on how careful we ought to be with this priceless resource 'water'. The same picture of neglect and interference is to be found worldwide. Our attitude to this valuable source of life seems to be one of contempt.

The political issue is of importance in that we have now indeed become each other's keeper, and we have to learn the lesson that this gift from nature deserves more respectful consideration than we have given it so far, and that we must not compound the present problems by further interference with life-giving resources, which tendency has already caused more than enough problems and illness. Every time I discuss this subject I am pleasantly surprised to discover how aware the majority of the public are of the dangers, and that they appear to demand a more sensible long-term approach. I have touched upon this subject in my lectures throughout the world and I always try to alert my audience to what is deemed necessary nowadays for the conservation of water, the development of its supply, its sewage collection and treatment and any improvements that can be effected to the environment as a whole.

Let us look at some investigations that have taken place concerning the conditions in the North Sea. Although some steps have already been taken, the water in the North Sea is far from what it should be. We will first consider the international meetings of scientists, the first of which was held in Bremen (West Germany) as long ago as 1984. This was followed by a conference in London in 1987 and the most recent one took place in the Hague (the Netherlands). Despite the attendance of eminent scientists at these international gatherings, the problems in the North Sea have hardly shown any sign of improvement. You may remember the recent epidemic that killed 16,000 seals, 60 per cent of which were washed ashore in the countries bordering the North Sea. We have been informed that this epidemic was due to a virus; this shows that the immune system of these delightful creatures was unable to protect them against this foreign invader. This, in turn, bears out the theory I

118

have adhered to for so many years, namely that the only protection against adverse environmental influences is to give more consideration to our immune system. These poor animals fell victim to such a sudden increase in pollution in the waters they have habitually thrived in that it strained their inborn immunity to breaking point.

At the second conference, held in London in 1987, we were led to believe that many important steps were currently under consideration, and yet, what has come of all these laudable plans? An investigation by Greenpeace showed that seven of the eight countries with responsibility for the North Sea environment have prepared plans in an effort to reduce the pollution by at least 50 per cent. I would imagine that it would be a frightening experience if we ever have a chance to take a look at the bottom of the North Sea when we consider the rubbish we feel free to dispose of in that body of water.

We have great expectations of the water in the world's seas, in that we hope that it can be of help in meeting the energy shortage. Yet we should give some consideration to the fact that pollution of the seas is expressed not only in atmospheric pollution; it also affects us physically. The choice of the word 'pollutant' is not only self-explanatory, but also merited. The actions of mankind have disturbed the marine environment and ecology and are also responsible for the damage done to its natural beauty.

Pollutants in the sea are introduced in several ways. Shipping and the careless dumping of oil must be major factors, together with the controversial issue of the dumping of waste material and the disposal of untreated sewage into the sea.

In a newspaper article earlier this year, I read that millions of lives are put at risk by bathing in the sea or by eating seafood that has been caught in polluted water; in many cases this pollution is caused by the disposal of raw sewage into the sea. A new report has since revealed the

119

strongest evidence for linking coastal pollution to disease. In this study it is claimed that a helping of oysters or mussels could contain a whole string of viruses, including the deadly hepatitis virus. If you intend to spend your annual holiday at a coastal resort, you should remember that children under five are specifically prone to such influences as they have not had the time to develop an immunity to local pollutants. This newspaper report also emphasised that, according to a report from a United States Marine Environment Action Group, it can no longer be denied that there may well be a link between pollution of the seas and the incidence of illness. The first report I mentioned was released on the same day that health campaigners unveiled plans for Britain's daily safe bathing times. Members of Friends of the Earth intend to co-operate with environmental health officers in monitoring sea-water samples taken around the clock and subsequently provide advice to visitors to Norfolk beaches on times when it is least likely to be harmful to bathe in the sea.

Professor Alistair MacIntyre of Aberdeen University, one of the twenty scientists involved in this survey, has rejected the government-supported theory that sunlight and solar radiation quickly destroy such dangerous compounds. He claims that even the AIDS virus may be able to survive in the sea longer than was previously thought.

Top scientists have also warned that Scottish lakes and rivers, already plagued by acid rain, are facing a new pollution disaster in the form of nitrates from cars, power stations and agriculture. This report is very interesting. Reading this article I felt compelled to look up the results of a survey conducted in 1983 in which my daughter was involved. She spent a great deal of time working for the Highlands River Purification Board and wrote an excellent paper which showed the situation as it was then. Considering that this survey was carried out seven years ago, I can only comment that there is, as yet, no sign of improvement in the situation.

In this paper, she noted that most of the freshwater rivers in the Scottish Highlands Board area were of high quality. However, the condition of the tidal inshore waters was much less satisfactory. The predominant cause of this was, and is, the discharge of untreated sewage from public authority sewage systems, particularly in the Highland region. At that time her particular concern was directed at the town of Inverness and surroundings. There she found a classic pollution indicating polyshaete capitella capitata. The Cromarty Firth was then also causing great concern, as a large number of organic pollutants were found there, which at that particular time was considered a worrying factor. The report identified the different pollutants and also discussed the influence of acid rain, and when I turned to the conclusion of that report and the account of the resulting discussions, I found that it was generally accepted by the River Purification Board that more emphasis must be given to its efforts to fight pollution. In order to conquer this pollution the emphasis must be directed to one of the most widely spread and harmful causes of pollution, i.e. acid rain.

The OECD (Organisation for Economic Co-operation and Development) has been very active in its efforts to control the acid-rain factor. This organisation concentrates on promoting economic co-operation in jointly combatting this polluting influence, and has achieved considerable public support. The question remains, however, as to whether the conditions currently laid down are stringent enough and whether sufficient attention is being paid to the serious danger acid rain spells to Western Europe. The list of areas affected by acid rain grows longer every year.

It is frightening to learn that in one small loch in Scotland acid rain has had such an influence on the fish that while they once used to be very clearly white, these fish are now turning blue. The scale of pollutants present in that particular loch make staggering reading and it has been clearly shown that they are a direct result of acid rain. Only careful research and international co-operation can reverse the tide and, together, we must find a way to counteract this dreadful damage that is being inflicted on nature.

In the Netherlands a motion was carried, way back in 1983, to bring down the 5,900 acid equivalent per hectare existing in 1980 to 3,000 acid equivalent per hectare. As yet, this objective has not been achieved and new mandates are under consideration to express the urgency felt about this source of pollution. It is not only trees that fall prey to acid rain; the quality of the water in the seas and rivers has deteriorated equally rapidly. In this context let us not overlook the erosion of our monuments and historic buildings caused by acid rain. We cannot fool ourselves any longer, because the time has come when we cannot deny that this damage also expresses itself in an increased tendency towards infections, in conjunction with the damage caused to the ozone layer.

People used to wonder about the exact meaning of the expression 'acid rain'. Unfortunately, this term has become familiar to most of us, but I maintain that it is somewhat misleading. We would do better to refer to it as 'acid deposition'. The transport of certain gas-forming products, as used in aerosols for example, will increase the acid deposits mainly through three elements: sulphur dioxide (SO_2), nitrogen oxide (NO) and ammonia (NH_3).

Sulphur dioxide is soluble in water, but it oxidises into sulphuric acid. Sulphur dioxide can be transformed into sulphur oxide and other products and this happens in the Netherlands at a rate of 40 per cent. Nitrogen oxide does not dissolve well in water and is often transformed into nitric acid (NO_3). A third of the acidity in the Netherlands can be attributed to the reactions to nitrogen oxide. Ammonia, being an alkaline component, neutralises the acids mentioned above, forming ammonia salts, which can make the air and rainwater less acid. However, when the deposition occurs on soil, ammonia and ammonia salts are partly transformed by micro-organisms into nitric acid. Because of the ammonia, the neutralised acids are freed once again and thus account for 25 per cent of the over-acidity in the Netherlands. Let us not become complacent in Britain, however, because similar statistics for this country are not much better. We should also bear in mind the fact that the pollution emanating from our car exhausts has a considerable influence in these statistics.

In a report written by Judy Stacey in *Today* magazine, the US government was urged to control and regulate the country's total toxic waste disposal by 73 per cent, its exposure to hazardous substances by 60 per cent and use of pesticides and herbicides by 52 per cent. So you will see that the situation existing in the United States is certainly no better than it is in Britain and other European countries.

The white cliffs of Dover are turning green because the ecological balance is being destroyed. This, in part, can be blamed on the Channel Tunnel works. It has been claimed by scientists that this phenomenon must be considered a geological tragedy.

Is it true that Britain is rapidly becoming one of the dirtiest, smelliest and noisiest countries — crying out for a cleaner environment? David Jones, in a newspaper article of Thursday, 29 March 1990, asks why we are not using the Government's powers in relation to environmental protection to the full. The so-called 'green policies' must be allowed to get to work. The output of nitrogen oxide has already rocketed to 2.48 billion tonnes. Levels of carbon monoxide are linked with diseases such as cancer and 26,926 water pollution incidents have been recorded in a single year, more than twice as many as in 1981, although only 327 of the culprits were taken to court. Why don't we put up more of a fight and register our dissatisfaction?

The EEC standards must be tightened up and be seen to be enforced. The seas would soon be considerably cleaner if more money was spent on the improvement of sewage treatment works. More access to environmental information is necessary in order to see and understand the full scale of these problems. Stories of coastal pollution have been scaring holidaymakers away, and the tourist boards, quite rightly, are worried and should put greater pressure on the authorities to clean up the environment. The enormous potential economic advantages of a flourishing domestic tourist industry should be evident from the fact that annual spending on foreign travel amounts to nearly £70 billion. What is happening to the beautiful holiday beaches of Great Britain? In the twenty years I have lived in Scotland I have seen a great decline in the cleanliness of the beaches around the Clyde. Our beautiful country has so much to offer, but why do we take it all for granted and shirk our individual responsibilities? If we see this wilful neglect of these gifts nature has endowed on us, should we not make it our business to make our voice heard?

In the spirit of this book I must stress how important sea-bathing can be for one's health. A female patient once consulted me after she had been told that she was suffering from an incurable oedema. I told her to bathe and exercise in the sea, and she could hardly believe it when she fully recovered from this condition. Because she took her daily exercise in the sea, her legs became completely normal again and she was once again able to relax her muscles. I have no doubt that our health will improve if we can bathe and swim in sea water and enjoy the benefits of the natural minerals contained therein, as well as enjoying its cleansing effects. It is quite a few years now since I gave this advice to a patient who thrived on the programme, but would I still dare to recommend this course of action in this day and age, knowing what I do about pollution? Similarly, I wonder how many patients would unquestionably follow my advice? Surely it is a wonderful sight to take a stroll on a lovely summer's day and see people enjoying the healing powers of the sea and breathing in the ozone-rich air. So, as you watch the beauty of a sunrise or sunset in all its glory . . . be reminded of our responsibilities. The majestic red haze from the sun reminds us of a new hope and a new age, evaluating our inheritance. Let it be ours to protect, to use and to respect.

Bibliography

Luc Cuyvers, *Het Beheer van onze zeëen*, Uitgeverij de Nederlandse Boekhandel, Antwerpen, Belgium, and Amsterdam, the Netherlands.

Marijke M. A. Brunt, *Milieubesparend Huishouden*, Uitgeverij Natuur en Milieu, Utrecht, the Netherlands.

David Kinnersley, *Troubled Water – Rivers, Politics and Pollution*, Hilary Shipman Limited, London, UK.

Dr Tine Kaayk, *Waterbehandeling*, Uitgeverij, Nederlandse Reformhuizen, the Netherlands.

Dr S. Flamm and Dr A. Hoff, *Wie Kneipp Kur?*, Paracelsus Verlag, Stuttgart, West Germany.

Dr Y. Hettema, C. *Waterbehandeling*, Uitgeverij W. P. van Stockum & Zn, Den Haag, the Netherlands.

Dr A. ten Haaf, *Hoge Darmspoelingen,* Ankh Hermes, Deventer, the Netherlands.

Dr Hans Moolenburgh, *Fluoride – The Freedom Fight*, Mainstream Publishing, Edinburgh, Scotland.

Ross Trattler ND, DO, *Better Health through Natural Healing*, Thorsons Publishing Group, Wellingborough, Northants.

Kitty Campion, *Handbook of Herbal Health*, Sphere Books Limited, London, UK, and Sydney, Australia.

Dr A. Vogel, *The Nature Doctor – A Manual of Traditional and Complementary Medicine*, Mainstream Publishing, Edinburgh, Scotland.

Dr Peter Mansfield and Jean Monro, *Chemical Children – How to Protect your Family from Harmful Pollutants*, Century Paperbacks, London, UK.